UNDERSTANDING ANTIEPILEPTIC DRUGS

Guiding You Through the Maze of Options

BERND POHLMANN-EDEN MD PHD

Professor of Neurology, Pharmacology, and Psychology
Director, Epilepsy Program Development
Member, Brain Repair Center
Dalhousie University
Halifax, Nova Scotia, Canada

BERNHARD J. STEINHOFF MD PHD

Medical Director and Executive Chief Physician, Epilepsy Clinic for Adults
Kork Epilepsy Centre, Epilepsiezentrum
Kork, Germany

Translation By Klaus C. Hofer

OXFORD
UNIVERSITY PRESS

OXFORD
UNIVERSITY PRESS

Oxford University Press is a department of the University of
Oxford. It furthers the University's objective of excellence in research,
scholarship, and education by publishing worldwide.

Oxford   New York
Auckland   Cape Town   Dar es Salaam   Hong Kong   Karachi
Kuala Lumpur   Madrid   Melbourne   Mexico City   Nairobi
New Delhi   Shanghai   Taipei   Toronto

With offices in
Argentina   Austria   Brazil   Chile   Czech Republic   France   Greece
Guatemala   Hungary   Italy   Japan   Poland   Portugal   Singapore
South Korea   Switzerland   Thailand   Turkey   Ukraine   Vietnam

Oxford is a registered trademark of Oxford University Press
in the UK and certain other countries.

Published in the United States of America by
Oxford University Press
198 Madison Avenue, New York, NY 10016

Library of Congress Cataloging-in-Publication Data
Pohlmann-Eden, Bernd, author.
Understanding antiepileptic drugs : guiding you through the maze of
options / by Bernd Pohlmann-Eden, Bernhard J. Steinhoff ; preface, Donald
Weaver ; translation, Klaus C. Hofer.—1st English edition.
    p. ; cm.
ISBN 978-0-19-935891-5 (alk. paper)
I. Steinhoff, Bernhard J., author.   II. Title.
[DNLM: 1. Anticonvulsants.   2. Epilepsy—drug therapy. QV 85]
RM322 615.7'84—dc23
2013051030

9 8 7 6 5 4 3 2 1
Printed in the United States of America
on acid-free paper

UNDERSTANDING
ANTIEPILEPTIC DRUGS

CONTENTS

PREFACE: FIRST ENGLISH EDITION

Epilepsy is the most frequent neurological disorder after cerebrovascular diseases. Medical treatment is the mainstay, with a wide range of therapeutic options that achieve seizure freedom or long-term remission in two-thirds of all people with epilepsy (PWE). It is critical to individualize and tailor the choice of drug to achieve the best treatment results and to keep the patient satisfied. This is particularly true with the first choice of antiepileptic drugs (AED), as almost half of all PWE become seizure free with the first AED and may stay on it for a long period of time.

Both authors have extensive experience in treating PWE and over time have appreciated the paramount importance of good compliance and a trusting relationship between patient and physician for a successful treatment outcome. The authors consider it key that the patient develop a deep understanding of the underlying epileptic process and the treatment options provided by each AED under discussion. Making the patient the "expert" of his or her disease will offer unique opportunities. Currently, PWE often get lost or "frustrated" by the detailed, difficult-to-understand information provided by the product monograph. In addition, a wide range of AEDs is now available, which may further increase the confusion of the patient, who may feel lost in a "jungle of options."

A decade ago, we therefore decided—as members of the AED committee of the German Epilepsy Society (a chapter of the International League against Epilepsy)—to publish a booklet with continuously updated and organized information on all available AEDs, which was easy to digest and understandable for patients, caregivers, nurses, nurse practitioners, family physicians, and other groups of health care professionals. This book is intended to provide a comprehensive overview of the efficacy profile of each AED, with a safety profile that addresses all organs. It is meant to enable the patient to better distinguish between rare and more frequent, or harmless and serious side effects. Mechanisms of action, as well as the role of slow release formulations and generic drugs, and special issues such as pregnancy are described in detail. This book was a huge success in Europe and has been very well received. The sixth German edition is on the way.

This first English edition targets people with epilepsy and their caregivers living in North America. All new antiepileptic drugs are presented in a clear fashion, including "orphan drugs" that recently have been approved either in Canada or the United States. By definition, these drugs are highly effective medications that apply to very rare ailments, and thus they have been subjected to an intentionally formal but relaxed approval process. In this way, rufinamide for the treatment of Lennox-Gastaut syndrome and stiripentol for the treatment of Dravet syndrome were officially introduced. In addition, the new antiepileptic drugs lacosamide and eslicarbazepine acetate are explained in a detailed and understandable format.

This book is the result of the excellent cooperation and critical support of many wonderful people. We would particularly like to thank Klaus C. Hofer, our translator, for his very professional, systematized approach, which has achieved a translation that accomplishes both "easy reading" and localization (transcultural aspect). Dr. Silke C. Eden initiated and coordinated all necessary steps of this process to arrive at a well-balanced and integrated result. We received substantial medical advice by our Canadian colleagues Dr. Mark Sadler, Dr. William Pryse-Phillips, and Dr. Donald Weaver, who, at this time president of Epilepsy Canada, also has written the preface to this book. Several health care professionals and colleagues involved in daily epilepsy care were asked to review the manuscript to ensure that the medical information is easy to understand and appropriate for laypersons. We particularly would like to thank family physician Dr. Gillian Achenbach, Epilepsy Coordinator Susan Rahey, Epilepsy Nurse Megan Williams, and Epilepsy Nurse Practitioner Karen Legg, who diligently accomplished the final editing of this manuscript. We are very thankful for any feedback and corrections with regard to this first English Edition.

We hope that this book will contribute to an improved communication between patients and physicians and ultimately will lead to better seizure control and quality of life for people with epilepsy.

Bernd Pohlmann-Eden
Halifax, Canada

Bernhard J. Steinhoff
Kehl-Kork, Germany

April 2014

PREFACE: FIFTH GERMAN EDITION

Dear Patient,

The intervals between the editions of our intentionally simplified and easily understandable reference book to guide through the maze of antiepileptic medications are getting shorter. In this case, it was just over two years. This is partially due to the popularity of the book's layout. This is especially pleasing, as patient-doctor cooperation is close to our hearts, as is the continuous monitoring of dynamic changes and the expansion of medicated treatment options for epilepsy. This edition has been completely reworked and updated. All new antiepileptic drugs are presented in a clear fashion, including the so-called orphan drugs, recently approved in Germany for the first time. By definition, these drugs are highly effective medications that apply to very rare ailments, and thus they have been subjected to an intentionally formal but relaxed approval process. In this way, rufinamide (Inovelon®) for the treatment of Lennox-Gastaut syndrome and stiripentol (Diacomit®) for the treatment of Dravet syndrome were officially introduced. In addition, the antiepileptic drug lacosamide, which serves as an add-on in the treatment of focal epilepsies for patients over 16 years old, is explained in a detailed and understandable format.

We address its therapeutic effect and side effect spectrum, as well as the available formats (tablets, syrup, and intravenous solution). Once again, we greatly appreciate your feedback if this fifth edition has satisfied the demand for easily understandable up-to-date information on antiepileptic medications. We look forward to your constructive criticism and recommendations to assure that this book retains its solid position in the family of medical consultation literature.

Bernd Pohlmann-Eden
Halifax, Canada

Bernhard J. Steinhoff
Kehl-Kork, Germany

Spring 2009

FOREWORD

The history of epilepsy is long, probably as ancient as that of man himself; it is a history of deities and demons, of spirits and curses—thus it is a story of human suffering and of medical ignorance. The history of treatments for epilepsy is equally long, with several thousand substances and procedures having been considered as potential treatments—ranging from the vile to the clever, and from bile to urine.

The earliest references to the treatment of epilepsy may be found in the Mesopotamian descriptions of *antasabbu* ("the falling disease") and in Ayurvedic writings of Asian Indian origin, dating to the fifth millennium BCE. During these ancient times, epilepsy ("the sacred disease") was regarded as an illness sent by the gods and thus was best treated through animal or human sacrifices, exorcisms, or participation in religious acts. *On the Sacred Disease*, written in 400 BCE, provides the first attempt at a scientific explanation for epilepsy. This treatise argued that seizures did not arise from evil spirits, but rather from an excess of "cold phlegm" secreted by the pituitary and accumulating in the cerebral ventricles. However, despite these early (but actually wrong) attempts to achieve a supposed scientific understanding of epilepsy, it remained a medical condition surrounded by superstition and mystique.

This preoccupation with superstition and mystique is reflected by the inadequate therapies of that ancient period. In primitive times, surgical therapies included trephining holes through the skull to release "evil humors." The ancients also employed a bizarre assortment of ad hoc "medical" therapies, ranging from rubbing the body of an epileptic with the genitals of a seal, to inducing sneezing at bedtime. In early Roman times, human blood was widely regarded as curative against the evil curse of epilepsy, and epileptics frequently sucked the blood of fallen gladiators or consumed powdered human skull (*cranum humanum* therapy).

By the Middle Ages, alchemy, astrology, and witchcraft were forming the "scientific" foundations of epilepsy therapy. The use of magical prayers and rituals was widespread; not surprisingly, hagiotherapy, a principle of treatment based on sacred objects and incantations to saints, flourished. To ward off evil spirits, necklaces and "anticonvulsion chains" made from the vertebrae of snakes were also popular. Other less spiritual remedies ranged from the use of stone amulets to grotesque therapies, such as the ingestion of dog bile or human urine. Plant-based therapy (phytotherapy) also flourished during the Middle Ages; almost every plant, shrub, or weed growing in the temperate forests of Europe was used to treat the "falling sickness."

During the subsequent Renaissance, medieval magical treatments for epilepsy were rejected by the medical profession in favor of so-called "rational" Galenic therapies, which included forced vomiting and bowel purging with simultaneous oral administration of peony extracts. In addition, a wide variety of rather toxic chemical substances (e.g., strychnine, curare, atropine, and quinine) were introduced as putative drug therapies for the suppression of seizures. Copper-based therapy also flourished during the Renaissance, and significant "therapeutic successes" were described; these reported successes with copper therapy led to other therapeutic attempts with lead, bismuth, tin, silver, iron, and mercury, thus giving rise to the concept of metallotherapy. There were also advances in the mechanistic understanding of epilepsy. The *Traite de l'epilepsie* by Samuel Tissot, for example, emerged as a source of intellectual illumination during the Renaissance. Tissot eloquently discussed how extracerebral disorders (e.g., kidney failure) and cerebral lesions (e.g., brain tumors) could produce seizures. Nevertheless, his work failed to influence therapy in a meaningful way, and the treatments of the Renaissance continued to be dominated by mystique—permitting charlatanism, superstition, and quackery to prosper. The description of King Charles II's death provides a comprehensive summary of the complexity and futility of seizure therapy during this time period:

> In 1685, the king fell backward and had a violent convulsion. Treatment for this seizure was begun immediately by a dozen physicians. He was bled to the extent of 1 pint from his right arm. Next, his shoulder was incised and cupped, depriving him of another 8 oz. of blood. After an emetic and two purgatives, he was given an enema containing antimony, bitters, rock salt, mallow leaves, violets, beet root, chamomile flowers, fennel seed, linseed, cinnamon, cardamom seed, saffron and aloes. The enema was repeated in 2 hours and another purgative was given. The king's head was shaved and a blister was raised on his scalp. A sneezing powder of hellebore root and one of cowslip flowers were administered to strengthen the king's brain. Soothing drinks of barley water, licorice and sweet almond were given, as well as extracts of mint, thistle leaves, rue, and angelica. For external treatment, a plaster of Burgundy pitch and pigeon dung was applied to the king's feet. After continued bleeding and purging, to which were added melon seed, manna, slippery elm, black cherry water, and dissolved pearls, the king's condition did not improve and, as an emergency measure, 40 drops of human skull extract were given to allay convulsions. Finally, bezoar stone was given. As the king's condition grew increasingly worse, the grand finale of Raleigh's antidote, pearl julep, and ammonia water were forced down the dying king's throat.

By the mid 1800s, the medical sciences were experiencing significant advances (e.g., anaesthesia, sterilization). Thus, the time was propitious for equally significant advances in the area of epileptology. Bromide therapy provided this much-needed advance, permitting epileptology to advance beyond the primitive quackeries of earlier times. By the early 1900s, meaningful advances in the medical treatment of epilepsy began to appear at a significant rate, including phenobarbital from Germany (in 1912) and phenytoin from the United States (in 1938). These two drugs heralded a flood of new and useful drugs for epilepsy throughout the remainder of the 1900s, a trend that has continued into the twenty-first century.

We are now a decade into the twenty-first century, and there are many effective drugs available for the treatment of seizure disorders. The optimal use of these agents is a partnership between the physician and the person with the seizure disorder. For people with seizures, a sound understanding of the drugs available to treat epilepsy enables them to be active participants in their own care and treatment. *Understanding Antiepileptic Drugs* by Bernd Pohlmann-Eden and Bernhard Steinhoff offers this understanding in a straightforward and readable fashion. Originally written in German, the English version affords a succinct and authoritative overview of drugs currently being used to treat epilepsy—with useful pearls of wisdom about each and every agent.

Donald F. Weaver
Director of Toronto Western Research Institute
at the University of Toronto, Canada

INTRODUCTION

A Guide for the Patient

As long-term members of the German Chapter of the International League against Epilepsy, we would like to share our experiences with antiepileptic medications and their side effects. These are observations that we further reviewed in consultation with a specially assembled board. This work was done in order to develop a handbook for patients, to help them actively participate in their treatment and, together with their doctor, to monitor and control possible side effects.

A medication completely free of side effects may never exist. Thus the patient and the treating physician must stay focused on possible side effects. Ongoing research and development of new pharmaceuticals aims to minimize side effects, but they may never be completely eliminated. Despite careful research and stringent controls, it will take years before accurate statements about side effects, especially long-term side effects, can be made. Side effects cause fear. This may be justified and beneficiary, as it heightens a sense of caution. However, unwarranted fears are frequently generated. Thus patients should recognize and differentiate the following: Unwarranted fears stem from lack of information, due to not understanding the actual side effects, which if misunderstood may lead to panic, or dramatization caused by prejudice. Justified fears instead are based on research-based knowledge about undesired medicinal effects and the probability of assumed side effects, or preexisting conditions, and so on. A strained relationship between the patient and the physician will always raise concerns and fears on the patient's side. It is hoped that this book will contribute to a trustful mutual and successful partnership between patient and physician.

PATIENT RECOMMENDATIONS

A Guide for the Patient

Upon completion of a thorough examination by the doctor, you should request a detailed explanation about possible side effects from the prescribed medication. Please read the product description carefully beforehand and write down any questions that may arise. During the consultation you should address all fears and concerns, even if they turn out to be groundless. Always insist on a conclusive answer. With the answers, new questions may arise that should be noted and discussed. This may become especially apparent if you are adjusting to a new or changed medication. All possible contraindications and interactions of different medications are as important, as is the question: What actions are required in this situation? Only on the basis of mutual trust can a good solution to the problem of side effects be effected. Your active participation in this process is as crucial as the work of the physician. Long-term epilepsy treatment facilities care for numerous patients with severe epilepsy, with prescribed high dosages of combinations of medications. Research has confirmed that patients under continuous medical supervision suffered no lasting medication-related side effects. Physicians are continuously learning about acute and long-term side effects. Their professional awareness on possible side effects has to grow constantly. It is mandatory that the physician acquire and maintain an up-to-date knowledge of all side effects.

This book informs about the side effects of the individual specific drugs (medications). The aim at the onset of any therapy is to manage with only one medication (monotherapy). Ideally, this should be one of the first choices, one that promises the best possible results. Only observations during the course of the therapy will show if you respond to the selected medication. The reason that a given medication is effective in some people but not effective in others, even though they are being treated for the same type of epilepsy, is still an open question. When treatment efforts with a single medication (monotherapy) fail, a combination of medications (combination therapy) may be required. Note that this approach may carry a higher risk of side effects than the monotherapeutic approach.

Close attention to these issues should be paid when discussing the individual medications. The primary objective with all medication treatments is to establish optimal blood levels through scheduled and timely administration of the medication. Failing to do so may lead to loss of treatment effect and may increase the risk of side effects.

ALCOHOL

We advise caution when consuming alcoholic beverages during treatment with antiepileptic medication. The effect of alcohol may possibly be amplified. In addition alcohol may promote the onset or frequency of seizures. A glass of beer or wine during special events is generally acceptable. However, hard liquors (whiskey, cocktails, etc.) should be avoided, as this may lead to a lower seizure threshold. As a motorist, you may risk losing your driver's license due to alcohol, and may endanger other motorists. In combination with antiepileptic medication, your driving abilities may be dangerously reduced.

CONTRACEPTION, PREGNANCY, AND BREAST FEEDING

Managing antiepileptic medication therapy in conjunction with family planning, during pregnancy, or while nursing a baby depends on your individual case, and the individual medications used. The basic rule always applies: Discuss this topic with your neurologist as well as your gynecologist before it becomes acute. All challenging situations should be resolved in consultation with a neurologist specialized in treating epileptic patients. It is of critical importance to consult your physician immediately to address a wanted pregnancy, or an already begun pregnancy. Only then can you be sure that all unique and known pregnancy-related issues with antiepileptic medications are adequately addressed. In addition to the consultation, early documentation of the progress of your pregnancy within the Europe-wide pregnancy registry EURAP (www.Eurap.de) is possible. This information contributes to the quality of consultations over the years, because the global consolidation of data to this topic continues to increase our knowledge.

The preferred course of action is monotherapy and minimal dosages. We hope that data from the pregnancy registry will soon enable us to consult more accurately on this important matter as we can today.

USER GUIDELINES

This book presents the most important antiepileptic medications currently in use. They are sorted by active ingredients and by their current trade names. You will learn about impact, area of application, and possible side effects currently known. The content is marked to allow you to determine when a physician or specialist should be consulted.

The basic rule stands: Severe side effects, be they frequent or rare, must always be quickly reported to a specialist (epileptologist).

The following notations mark how we classify side effects:

- *I = Information: Harmless side effects → Part of the initial medical consultation, no consequences within 14 days.*
- *FP = Family physician: frequent/rare less severe side effects → requires contact with your physician as soon as possible.*
- *S = needs specialist consultation.*
- *P = → Immediately contact your physician within hours of the incident.*
- *ED = Emergency department: in any case of serious adverse effect.*

GENERIC DRUGS

What Are They? Are There Risks?

A Guide for the Patient

If your doctor, your drug plan, or your pharmacist suggests that cost-efficient medications containing the same active substances as the "brand name" product are available, then, in most likelihood, they are speaking about a "generic drug." Generic drugs are approved drugs that are precise replicas of their original predecessors. In comparison, "brand name" drugs have gone through complex development and testing processes to gain approval. With this approval the original drugs also obtained patent protection for a given time. When this original patent protection expires, other qualified drug companies can obtain a license to produce and market these replications. These replications are known as generic drugs. Generic drugs are usually less expensive and may offer a different capsule or tablet casing structure, although the active substances they contain and the dosages are identical. Generic drug approval requires that the active agents (after oral administration) fall within an 80–125% range of the original product. This is also known as "bioequivalent." In many cases, generic drugs offer economic advantages, while offering a medically equivalent solution. This applies especially during the initial drug adjustment phase. Some members of the professional community expressed concerns when switching patients from original drugs to generic drugs after seizures have stopped. All other possible variations should be thoroughly discussed with your specialist.

SLOW (OR CONTROLLED) RELEASE DRUGS

What Are They? Are There Risks?

A Guide for the Patient

Antiepileptic medicated treatment therapy is usually a permanent treatment decision. It is therefore essential to focus on and establish optimal tolerance. Some antiepileptic medications will be absorbed quickly by the body after administration. This may result in temporary peak concentrations of the active agents in your blood. However, they are not necessary for long-term effectiveness and may trigger side effects. This can be avoided through the so-called slow release technology of your medication. "Slow release" or "controlled release" means that the release of the active agents contained in your medication is slowed in a controlled manner. This allows for consistent drug levels in the bloodstream over the duration of the treatment and prevents drug peaks in the bloodstream, which could trigger side effects.

Among the antiepileptic medications available as slow release form are carbamazepine and valproic acid. The absence of slow release forms among other antiepileptic medications does not mean that these are lacking when compared to the above-mentioned medications. Not all antiepileptic drugs require a release edition.

ORPHAN DRUGS

What Are They? Are There Risks?

A Guide for the Patient

This term originated in the Anglo-American literature. It refers to medications approved to treat the so-called orphan diseases, which are defined as diseases that occur so rarely that development, testing, and approval of new medications, in the numbers customarily required, is not possible. An additional problem is that many of these diseases are quite severe and urgently need new and effective therapy solutions. As a result, the Orphan Drug Act was created in 1983, to enable the development and approval of such medications. So far, more than 6,000 rare diseases qualifying as orphan diseases have been identified. The qualification criteria for the status of "medication for the treatment of rare diseases" may be based on epidemiological arguments (no more than 5 patients within 10,000) as well as economical arguments (economically not feasible).

Medications for the treatment of rare diseases may become subject to a more relaxed approval process. Required are controlled observations that point to a high probability of effectiveness, and acceptable tolerance. This assures that the known risks are within an acceptable range.

When approved, the developer receives exclusive marketing rights for the "approved indication" of this drug for ten years. Generally, this time-limited approval is tied to additional responsibilities, which mainly encompass detailed documentation and ongoing research to allow for better understanding of effectiveness and tolerance.

The following paragraph refers to European countries only; these medications are not available in Canada. The first release of orphan drugs for treatment of epilepsy in 2007 and 2008 were rufinamide (Inovelon®) and stiripentol (Diacomit®). These medications were used for treating Lennox-Gastaut syndrome (rufinamide) and Dravet syndrome (Stiripentol). The approval of these two medications required that only caregivers who are specialists in the treatment of epilepsy may prescribe these drugs.

SPECIFIC PROFILES OF ANTIEPILEPTIC DRUGS (IN ALPHABETICAL ORDER)

Carbamazepine | How Does It Work? What Are the Side Effects?

Dear patient,
Your doctor has prescribed carbamazepine for the treatment of your epilepsy.

Based on years of observations in the management of epilepsies, we want to inform you about the effects and side effects of this medication. In addition to the standard product description that came with your medication, we share with you our expertise in a simple and understandable format. The information here is not intended to replace the product description that came with your medication. Instead, you should read it thoroughly to filter out information that pertains to you. This guide provides solid advance information to initiate a detailed consultation with your doctor.

HOW DOES CARBAMAZEPINE WORK? WHAT IS THE CORRECT DOSAGE?

Carbamazepine was introduced in 1963 as the first tricyclic antiepileptic medication. It stabilizes the electrical excitability of neural membranes. As such, sudden discharges of multiple neurons occur less frequently, or not at all. Carbamazepine suppresses the spread of excitation to neighboring regions of the brain.

The active ingredients are absorbed into the gastrointestinal tract within two to eight hours. This varies greatly from patient to patient. Only one-third of carbamazepine binds to blood proteins. Through the metabolic activity within the liver, additional antiepileptic substances (epoxides) are built, which also suppress seizures, but which may also be responsible for some side effects. Carbamazepine belongs to the group of enzyme inducers. As such, it accelerates the metabolic rate of the liver. The effectiveness of carbamazepine may become reduced during the initial adjustment phase, requiring a subsequent increase in dosage. Frequently, significant interactions with other substances, which are also processed by the liver, are observed. These include antiepileptic medications such as phenytoin and phenobarbital. The effectiveness of common supplementary prescriptions such as Warfarin® and related psychopharmacological drugs may also be impeded. Also, vitamin D and sexual hormones may diminish. The recommended dosage of carbamazepine is 1–20 mg/kg of body weight. The daily dosage varies individually between 600 mg and 2,400 mg but may, on occasion, be more. Tablets are available in units of 200 mg, and in addition, 200 mg and 400 mg as controlled release formulations. There are also chewable tablets of 100 mg and 200 mg and a suspension of 100 mg/5 ml.

The amount of carbamazepine required for treatment depends on the severity of the illness as well as the weight of the patient and metabolic aspects. Slow initiation with a smaller dosage improves individual drug tolerance. Dosage then can be stepped up gradually. The individual dosage, suitable for your type of seizure, must be carefully determined by your doctor over the course of several visits. Therefore, don't become discouraged if a dosage increase becomes necessary and if, during the initial treatment phase, the desired results do not occur immediately. Do not discontinue your medication from one day to the next, even if you are free of seizures. You would only risk new seizures. If the medication has not shown the anticipated results when reasonably expected, your physician may prescribe a different product. Carbamazepine then must be tapered off gradually. The timing and alternate medication shall be discussed with your doctor. In general, the risk of recurring seizures may be greater during this transition phase.

WHAT DO WE TREAT WITH CARBAMAZEPINE, AND HOW EFFECTIVE IS IT?

Carbamazepine is among the best-researched antiepileptic drugs in terms of effectiveness and side effects. It is frequently prescribed for the treatment of partial seizures, with or without loss of consciousness, as well as secondarily generalized clonic-tonic seizures. This medication has no or little effect on primary generalized epileptic seizures (such as age-related absence seizures), atonic seizures, or myoclonic seizures; it may even intensify, or trigger, these.

For between 70% and 80% of epilepsy patients who respond to carbamazepine, a long-term and significant reduction, or even a complete suppression, of seizures can be expected.

WHAT DO YOU NEED TO KNOW ABOUT THE SIDE EFFECTS OF CARBAMAZEPINE?

Brain and Psyche

During the initial adjustment phase, or during an increase of the dosage, patients frequently report fatigue, sedation, tiredness, and drowsiness (I/S). Frequently, these symptoms start to disappear after days, or a few weeks. In the event of dizziness, ask a relative or friend to check if your eyes are "shaking." Your doctor calls this "nystagmus" and will gladly explain how to diagnose it. Nystagmus may indicate a slight over-dosage. If the above-mentioned side effects occur frequently, or last longer than expected, consult your doctor. The doctor may then request a blood test to evaluate your carbamazepine dosage. Improvements have often been achieved by simply reducing the dosage, or by adjusting the schedule of administration over the course of the day. You may be concerned that the medication could interfere with your physical, as well as your intellectual (FP/S), performance. Current discussion in the scientific literature on this is inconclusive. Some studies claimed deterioration in concentration ability, while others found that carbamazepine had no impact on intellectual performance. It important to keep in mind that epileptic discharges themselves, or seizure, can temporarily reduce both memory function and concentration.

In individual cases, the antiepileptic medication may not be the primary cause for memory impairment. Should you feel that your physical or intellectual performance is impeded due to carbamazepine, consult your doctor. Perhaps a minor dosage adjustment may provide relief (I/S).

Allergies and Skin

Immediately report noticeable changes to your skin, as well as itching and/or a fever (FP/S). Between 8% and 10% of patients may show allergic reactions to carbamazepine. These may not be immediately apparent, but could appear weeks after commencing treatment. In this case, a change of medication may be the only solution.

Blood

Occasional changes in your blood count can be found. In most cases, a harmless reduction in white cells is observed. To be sure, your doctor will monitor your blood count during treatment with carbamazepine, especially during the initial adjustment phase.

Bone

Reduced bone density may occur due to the effect on enzyme induction of carbamazepine (see under Additional Information) (S).

Gastrointestinal Tract and Internal Organs

Liver damage, even after years of treatment, is not expected. An increase in the gamma-GT value only indicates increased liver activity. With other values in the normal range, a double or triple increase of the gamma-GT value is insignificant and may not indicate illness (FP/S). It is extremely rare for hepatitis to occur. Should your skin turn yellow, however, or if nausea, loss of appetite, or fatigue occurs, visit your doctor immediately.

Heart

We do not expect side effects on the heart. Rarely, cases of heart block have been reported. In the presence of known heart disease, consult your physician, as the risk may be increased.

Interaction with Other Drugs

Carbamazepine is an enzyme inducer that accelerates the metabolic rate of the liver (resulting in the above described increase in the enzyme gamma-GT). Therefore, the serum levels of other antiepileptic drugs and of other drugs that are given because of indications other than epilepsy may fall. This can be clinically relevant if the effects of these drugs are not as expected. A dose change may be necessary (FP/S).

Additional Information

Only rarely do patients complain about the following, mostly harmless side effects: conjunctivitis, visual disturbance, or lens blurring. If these should occur, it is recommended to check the intraocular pressure (especially with glaucoma). Equally rare are nausea, loss of appetite, and irregularities within the gastrointestinal tract. A gentle introduction of the medication usually prevents (FP/S) this. Only in individual cases were irregularities in kidney function, composition of electrolytes, sexual problems, or weight increase observed. As noted above, carbamazepine is an enzyme inducer that accelerates the metabolic rate of the liver (resulting in the above described increase in gamma-GT). Long-term treatment may induce shortages of trace elements and reduction of hormones and vitamins as the result of the accelerated metabolism. Typical side effects resulting from shortages of trace elements are reduced bone density, nightly cramps in the thighs and calves, and pain in the soles of the feet. In this case, a change of medication may be considered (FP/S). A careful evaluation of risk and benefit in the individual case is now required. It should be noted that these symptoms may not only be due to the medication.

Contraception, Pregnancy, and Breast Feeding

As carbamazepine is metabolized in the liver, it increases the metabolic activity in the liver. This may lead to a higher rate of breakdown of other medications, possibly including the hormone-based agents in the contraceptive pill. This means that prevention of an unwanted pregnancy, managed by the contraceptive pill, is not certain while taking carbamazepine. Your doctor or gynecologist may, in that case, recommend other forms of contraception. Epilepsy, even if not treated with antiepileptic drugs, carries a very small risk of birth deformity. It is important to know that the risk of a birth defect due to carbamazepine therapy differs only marginally from the risk in untreated epilepsy patients. As the event of a major seizure (such as grand mal with fall and unconsciousness) presents a danger to your unborn child, the regularly scheduled administration of your medication during pregnancy is of special importance.

Today, early diagnostics are available to identify suspected birth defects. Your physician may, for example, request a special ultrasound test and a blood examination, to identify possible indicators of congenital deformities of the spine. These are assumed to occur more frequently than normal during carbamazepine therapy. Recent reports suggest that carbamazepine performs better than other antiepileptic drugs during pregnancy. Amniocentesis can provide a more precise answer in questionable cases. Your physician can tell you whether such a test is needed and, if so, when it should be scheduled.

We have now extensively informed you about the rare but possible side effects of carbamazepine. You should be aware that your doctor selected this medication as it presents the best possible treatment for your epilepsy, with the minimum of side effects.

Success with carbamazepine therapy is only possible if you take the medication as scheduled. Only in this way will you avoid large fluctuations of the drug in your blood. Once full dosage has been established and maximum blood levels have been reached, the rate of seizures should go down. If the frequency of seizures continues, you should seek the advice of your epilepsy specialist.

Clobazam

Dear patient,
  Your doctor has prescribed clobazam for the treatment of your
epilepsy. Based on years of observations in the management of epi-
lepsies, we want to inform you about the effects and side effects of
this medication. In addition to the standard product description
that came with your medication, we share with you our expertise
in a simple and understandable format. The information here is
not intended to replace the product description that came with
your medication. Instead, you should read it thoroughly to filter
out information that pertains to you. This guide provides solid
advance information to initiate a detailed consultation with your
doctor.

HOW DOES CLOBAZAM WORK?
WHAT IS THE CORRECT DOSAGE?

Clobazam belongs to the group of benzodiazepines. Other examples of benzodiazepines are diazepam, clonazepam, and loraz-
epam. Benzodiazepines are often used as emergency drugs in
status epilepticus, that is, a condition when epileptic seizures do
not stop and require emergency treatment. In chronic epilepsy
treatment, benzodiazepines are not frequently used. Why is that

the case? Although benzodiazepines have a very high efficacy against epileptic activity, their main disadvantages are sedating effects and the risk of addiction. That means that under chronic treatment conditions one often has to increase the dose in order to maintain the antiepileptic effect that declines over time. In addition, if the drug is to be discontinued, withdrawal symptoms including seizures may result. Both the sedating properties and the problem of tolerance and addiction may occur also with clobazam. However, compared to other benzodiazepines, the potential drawbacks are less pronounced so that clobazam is the only benzodiazepine that is widely used for chronic epilepsy treatment.

All benzodiazepines act by enhancing GABA (gamma-aminobutyric acid). GABA is a neurotransmitter with general inhibitory and calming properties in the brain. Therefore benzodiazepines not only have antiepileptic effects but also anxiolytic (anxiety-relieving) and hypnotic properties.

Clobazam is licensed in most parts of Europe and in Canada for the add-on use in patients with epilepsy. In the United States, it is labeled as an orphan drug for use in Lennox-Gastaut syndrome, a very severe and usually difficult-to-treat form of epilepsy.

The daily dosage of clobazam, in adults, usually starts with 5 mg to 15 mg per day, distributed according to a twice-daily dosing regimen. A gradual increase up to 80 mg may be necessary and possible. In children below 2 years, the initial dose is 0.5 mg to 1 mg/ kg/day; in older children, it is 5 mg per day, which may be increased at 5-day intervals to a maximum of 40 mg per day. Clobazam is distributed as white divisible tablets that contain 10 mg.

WHAT DO WE TREAT WITH CLOBAZAM, AND HOW EFFECTIVE IS IT?

Clobazam has been investigated in seven large clinical trials. Furthermore, there is a lot of evidence from several case series in differing epilepsy syndromes and age groups. Clobazam was shown to be effective both against focal and generalized seizures. In the United States, it is labeled for use in Lennox-Gastaut syndrome, a characteristic epilepsy syndrome mainly with drop attacks and generalized tonic-clonic (grand mal) seizures.

WHAT DO YOU NEED TO KNOW ABOUT THE SIDE EFFECTS OF CLOBAZAM?

Brain and Psyche

The most common side effects of clobazam are drowsiness, dizziness, and fatigue. Side effects that also occurred more often than in 1% of patients were gait disturbance, nervousness, behavior disorder, hostility, and blurred vision. However, the frequency of those latter adverse events is very low.

Of course, you should contact your physician (FP/S) in case of such adverse events. Usually he or she will decrease the dose or distribute it in another way in order to improve tolerability.

Allergies and Skin

Major allergic reactions are very rare; however, skin reactions when starting treatment may occur very occasionally and may even need emergency consultation (ED).

After initiation of the therapy (7th–10th day), rashes similar in appearance to that of measles may occur (FP/S). These are generally harmless and disappear when the dosage is reduced. Discontinuation of the medication is rarely required. The transition to more severe allergic reaction is indicated by the appearance of blisters on the skin and fever. If this happens, you must immediately consult your doctor (FP/S/ED).

Blood

Nothing known.

Bone

Nothing known.

Liver, Pancreas, and Kidneys

Nothing known.

Heart

Nothing known.

Interactions with Other Drugs

Most studies did not show clinically relevant interactions with other drugs. However, it has been reported that clobazam may increase the serum levels of carbamazepine, phenytoin, valproate, and phenobarbital. Alcohol increases the serum levels of clobazam. Serum levels of clobazam decrease slightly if carbamazepine, phenytoin, Phenobarbital, and valproic acid are co-administered.

Additional Information

In rare instances, dryness of mouth, constipation, loss of appetite, nausea, dizziness, muscle weakness, disorientation, and tiredness have been observed. Such a clinical situation would require you to contact the specialist or the emergency department (S/ED). In case of an overdose and intoxication, drowsiness, confusion, and reduced muscle reflexes are the main features. In severe cases, respiratory insufficiency, reduced blood pressure and heart rate, sedation, and coma may occur (ED).

Contraception, Pregnancy, and Breast Feeding

Clobazam does not have a clinically significant effect on the efficacy of the contraceptive pill. Clobazam, as all minor tranquilizers, may increase the risk of fetal deformities. However, the data concerning clobazam are not extensive. Clobazam passes into mother's breast milk. It may happen that fatigue and weaker sucking of the child is observed. In such cases, you should contact the specialist (S) and discuss with him whether you must discontinue to breast feed—of course gradually, to avoid withdrawal symptoms.

We have now thoroughly informed you about the rare but possible side effects of clobazam. You should be aware that your doctor selected this medication because it currently presents the best possible treatment for your epilepsy, with minimal side effects.

Successful clobazam therapy is only possible if you take the medication as directed. Only in this way will you avoid large fluctuations of the drug in your blood. Once full dosage has been established and maximum blood levels have been reached, the rate of seizures should go down. If this is not the case, you should seek the advice of your epilepsy specialist immediately.

Eslicarbazepine
Acetate
How Does
It Work?
What Are
the Side
Effects?

Dear patient,
  Your doctor has prescribed eslicarbazepine acetate for the treatment of your epilepsy. Eslicarbazepine acetate was approved in 2009 and was labeled as add-on treatment for focal seizures with or without secondary generalization, in patients 16 years or older in most European countries and more recently (November 2013) also in the US. Its approval in Canada is expected shortly. Due to the relatively short period since its release, the full scope of clinical effects and side effects will not be known for the next few years. The information here is not intended to replace the product description that came with your medication. Instead, you should read it thoroughly as well, to filter out important and less important information that pertains to you. This guide provides solid advance information to initiate a detailed consultation with your doctor.

HOW DOES ESLICARBAZEPINE ACETATE WORK? WHAT IS THE CORRECT DOSAGE?

Eslicarbazepine acetate, chemically seen, is a close relative of the well-established antiepileptic medication carbamazepine and the antiepileptic compound oxcarbazepine. Compared to carbamazepine, eslicarbazepine acetate undergoes a different metabolization, which may result in a better tolerability. Compared to oxcarbazepine, after metabolization of eslicarbazepine acetate a higher proportion of a product is found that has a preferential brain penetration and a particularly high efficacy without the potential tolerability problems that oxcarbazepine induces prior to metabolization. Thus, theoretically eslicarbazepine actetate should have some advantages in efficacy and tolerability. Whether or not this is true in the treatment of patients needs to be confirmed.

Eslicarbazepine acetate stabilizes and reduces the electrical tension on the neural membranes and as such reduces the probability of epileptic seizures. The individually required dosage of eslicarbazepine acetate differs from patient to patient. It depends on the severity of the disease, the weight of the patient, and metabolic issues. By slowly introducing the medication and gradually increasing the dosage to the desired level, you can significantly improve its tolerance. The individually suitable dosage, to treat your type of seizures, must be determined by your doctor over several appointments. Patience is required, as metabolization takes time. In view of the way in which eslicarbazepine acetate is metabolized, a once daily administration is recommended. In general, the daily dosage for adults ranges between 400 mg and 1,200 mg. In individual cases, it may be helpful to increase this dosage further in order to achieve optimal response. This should be discussed with your doctor on an individual basis. The medication is currently available as a divisible tablet in dosage units of 800 mg.

WHAT DO WE TREAT WITH ESLICARBAZEPINE ACETATE, AND HOW EFFECTIVE IS IT?

Eslicarbazepine acetate is used in the treatment of patients with partial and secondarily generalized tonic-clonic seizures (grand mal). In three randomized placebo-controlled trials, eslicarbazepine acetate was added to a preexisting baseline medication in adults with difficult-to-treat focal epilepsies. A statistically significant decrease in seizure frequency was shown for 800 mg and 1,200 mg but not for 400 mg, which showed a trend toward better efficacy; 800 mg and 1,200 mg were also significantly more effective than placebo concerning change in partial seizure frequency.

WHAT DO YOU NEED TO KNOW ABOUT THE SIDE EFFECTS OF ESLICARBAZEPINE ACETATE?

Brain and Psyche

During the initial treatment stage, when the daily dosage of eslicarbazepine acetate is gradually increased to the target level, symptoms such as dizziness, fatigue, and an unsteady gait may occur. In the event of dizziness, ask a relative or friend to check if your eyes are "shaking." Your doctor calls this "nystagmus" and will gladly explain how to diagnose it. Nystagmus may indicate a slight over-dosage. If the above symptoms don't go away, contact your family doctor immediately. If the symptoms intensify, contact your epilepsy specialist immediately. Generally, most of these annoying but usually harmless symptoms disappear soon after the adjustment phase, or after a minor dosage correction. Patients who are being treated with antiepileptic drugs occasionally report impairment of physical and intellectual properties. Neuropsychological studies have so far not identified a negative impact of eslicarbazepine acetate on intelligence, memory, or attention capacity. However, we cannot fully exclude the possibility of an individual occurrence. In the event that you suspect that this is the case with you, you should immediately consult a specialist or family physician (FP/S). Perhaps a small adjustment in your dosage will bring relief.

Allergies and Skin

Should you notice changes to your skin, itching, or fever (FP/S), which might be part of an allergic reaction, see your family doctor immediately or go to the nearest emergency department (although the clinical trials did not give evidence for an elevated risk for allergies and skin reactions so far).

Blood

Nothing known.

Bone

Nothing known.

Gastrointestinal Tract and Internal Organs

Gastrointestinal side effects are rare. Nausea and vomiting were occasionally observed. Diarrhea, obstipation, and abdominal pain were reported in single cases, but with a frequency that did almost not differ from that observed with placebo. A slow introduction to the medication may ease or even eliminate these effects.

Liver damage is not expected, even after years of treatment. Increases of two- and threefold of the liver enzyme gamma-GT have been observed, but this appears to be no reason for concern. These readings merely indicate the metabolic activity. Should you notice yellow skin color tone, exhaustion, nausea, or loss of appetite, these may be indicators of liver failure, occurring in very rare cases. Please seek professional help immediately (FP/S/ED). It is not yet clear if eslicarbazepine acetate may cause lowered blood sodium levels, which occasionally occurs with carbamazepine and oxcarbazepine. Studies so far did not show an elevated risk. However, due to the chemical relationship, we would suggest not to exclude generally that nausea and fatigue also may be due to lowered blood sodium levels. Thus your doctor will regularly monitor the electrolyte levels in your blood.

Heart

Nothing known.

Interactions with Other Drugs

Eslicarbazepine acetate is a mild enzyme inductor. As such, it accelerates the metabolic rate of the liver. However, the extent of the enzyme induction is significantly less than that with common antiepileptic drugs of similar characteristics. We cannot exclude the possibility that after a long-term therapy a shortage of micronutrients (trace elements), hormones, and vitamins may be noticed, due to the accelerated degradation. Stay alert for symptoms of these deficiencies. Indicators may be reduced bone density, cramps in the calf, and pain in the sole of the foot. In selected cases, a change in medication may be considered. This requires a careful review of the benefits versus risk relationship. It must be noted that the above-mentioned symptoms may not always stem either partially or fully from the medication (FP/S). Again, we want to bring to your attention that eslicarbazepine acetate is a new medication; as such, not all side effects are yet known. You should therefore discuss all unwanted physical and mental symptoms with your physician, including those that are not noted on the product description.

Contraception, Pregnancy, and Breast Feeding

Eslicarbazepine acetate does not accelerate the metabolic activity of the liver in the same fashion as other antiepileptic drugs.

However, it may still critically affect the contraceptive protection provided by the birth control pill. Epilepsy, even if not treated with antiepileptic drugs, carries a slight risk of fetal deformity. This risk is not increased if treated with only one antiepileptic drug. Animal tests have not indicated potential damage to fetal development. However, we always recommend early diagnostics to check on the healthy development of your child. If you become pregnant while already on eslicarbazepine acetate, you should not discontinue the medication on your own accord, as this could lead to an increase in seizures, presenting a greater harm to your baby than eslicarbazepine acetate itself. Consult a specialist immediately, and discuss further course of action.

We have now thoroughly informed you about the rare but possible side effects of eslicarbazepine acetate. You should be aware that your doctor selected this medication because it currently presents the best possible treatment for your epilepsy, with minimal side effects.

Successful eslicarbazepine acetate therapy is only possible if you take the medication as directed. Only in this way will you avoid large fluctuations of the drug in your blood. Once full dosage has been established and maximum blood levels have been reached, the rate of seizures should go down. If this is not the case, you should seek the advice of your epilepsy specialist immediately.

Ethosuximide | How Does It Work? What Are the Side Effects?

Dear patient,
  Your doctor has prescribed ethosuximide for the treatment of your epilepsy.
  Based on years of observations in the management of epilepsies, we want to inform you about the effects and side effects of this medication. In addition to the standard product description that came with your medication, we share with you our expertise in a simple and understandable format. The information here is not intended to replace the product description that came with your medication. Instead, you should read it thoroughly to filter out information that pertains to you. This guide provides solid advance information to initiate a detailed consultation with your doctor.

HOW DOES ETHOSUXIMIDE WORK? WHAT IS THE CORRECT DOSAGE?

The acting agent ethosuximide was introduced in 1952 to be used for the treatment of epilepsy (absence seizures). It was developed as an effective medication with few side effects. It is used for the treatment of a specific group of generalized seizures (absence seizures).

It stabilizes the electrical activity on the neural membranes and as such reduces the electrical activity. Due to its high effectiveness and easily manageable side effects, this medication has remained the primary choice for the treatment of the above named seizure types, for nearly 50 years after its introduction. The recommended therapeutic dosage for adults is 15 mg/kg of body weight, and for children 20 mg/kg of body weight. The general tablet strength is 250 mg. Ethosuximide is also available as a syrup (250 mg/5 ml).

WHAT DO WE TREAT WITH ETHOSUXIMIDE, AND HOW EFFECTIVE IS IT?

Ethosuximide is highly effective in absence seizures. Up to 80% of patients will be free of seizures with ethosuximide. Even in other forms of absence seizures accompanied by grand-mal seizures, 50% percent of all cases showed effectiveness with this treatment. Ethosuximide is also used successfully to control age-related epilepsies such as the so-called myoclonic-astatic petit mal seizures. This has been observed when ethosuximide was prescribed as a medication of second choice.

WHAT DO YOU NEED TO KNOW ABOUT THE SIDE EFFECTS OF ETHOSUXIMIDE?

Brain and Psyche

Fatigue, headaches, dizziness, labored movements, irritability, and sensitivity to light (photophobia) are occasional and mostly temporary (F/S). This is all in exchange for an almost complete and immediate relief from seizures. In rare cases, psychotic episodes (schizophrenia-like) or states of confusion occur. Such side effects may require the discontinuation of the medication.

Allergies and Skin

Rarely does ethosuximide lead to vascular inflammation. In such cases, immediate consultation with a specialist is required.

Look out for changes in the skin! Occasionally, allergic skin reactions (itchy redness and nodules) appear and, though unrelated to the dosage, may force a discontinuation of ethosuximide (P/S). In the event of very rare but serious skin disorders (i.e., development of enlarging blisters), consult your doctor immediately (FP/S) or go right away to the emergency department.

Blood

Ethosuximide may, in extremely rare cases, lead to changes in the blood cell count. These are mostly dependent on dosage and don't require a discontinuation of the medication. Principally, regular blood tests (FP) are recommended (monthly for the first 3 months, then if free of seizures, two times annually).

Bone

Nothing known.

Gastrointestinal Tract and Internal Organs

Digestive issues are rare. Symptoms may include nausea, vomiting, loss of appetite, loss of weight, diarrhea, and hiccups (I/FP/S). These effects frequently vanish a few days after treatment has commenced and are treatable with common medications. Extra caution is warranted in case of a preexisting liver disorder.

Interactions with Other Drugs

Clinically relevant interactions are not known.

Contraception, Pregnancy, and Breast Feeding

Although ethosuximide does not impact the serum concentrations of other medications, we cannot completely rule it out. As such, oral contraceptive protection cannot be guaranteed, and medical consultation is recommended. With low dosages and maintained low blood serum levels of ethosuximide, no birth defects have been observed with children whose mothers were treated with low dosages. With larger dosages and elevated serum plasma concentrations, and in combinations with phenytoin, occasional birth defects were reported. Ethosuximide carries into mother's milk and as such could lead to toxic symptoms in the nursing infant. The recommendation is to reduce the dosage of ethosuximide within the serum, especially in cases without grand mal risk, between the onset of pregnancy and completion of breast feeding. If there is no grand mal risk, and you only suffer from absences, discontinuation of ethosuximide prior to pregnancy and breast feeding may be considered.

We have now extensively informed you about the rare but possible side effects of ethosuximide. You should be aware that your doctor selected this medication as it presents the best possible treatment for your epilepsy, while carrying the least amount of side effects.

Success with ethosuximide therapy is only possible if you take the medication as scheduled. Only in this way will you avoid large fluctuations of the drug in your blood. Once full dosage has been established and maximum blood levels have been reached, the rate of seizures should go down. If the frequency of seizures continues, you should seek the advice of your epilepsy specialist.

Felbamate

How Does
It Work?
What Are
the Side
Effects?

Dear patient,
Your doctor has prescribed felbamate for the treatment of your epilepsy.

Based on years of observations in the management of epilepsies, we want to inform you about the effects and side effects of this medication. In addition to the standard product description that came with your medication, we share with you our expertise in a simple and understandable format. Felbamate was approved in Canada and the United States in 1993 and in Europe in 1995. It is only available through a special access program due to its potential side effects (see section on side effects). Approval meanwhile is usually limited to treatment of Lennox-Gastaut syndrome, a specific epileptic disorder that is difficult to treat and mainly is characterized by drop attacks and generalized tonic-clonic seizures (grand mal). Based on extensive observations since then, we have accumulated comprehensive knowledge about its effects and side effects. The information here is not intended to replace the product description that came with your medication. Instead, you should read it thoroughly to filter out information that pertains to you. This guide provides solid advance information to initiate a detailed consultation with your doctor.

HOW DOES FELBAMATE WORK?
WHAT IS THE CORRECT DOSAGE?

The composition of felbamate does not compare to other anti-epileptic medication. The mechanisms of action are not entirely understood, but it has an effect on inhibitory transmitter GABA (gamma-aminobutyric acid) receptor binding sites. It may also work as a receptor antagonist against excitatory binding sites.

Most studies report adult daily dosages between 1,200 and 3,600 mg. Children are treated with dosages ranging from 15 to 45 mg per kg of bodyweight. The recommended dosages correspond to the weight/mg ratios. The individually required and tolerable dosage must be determined and fixed by the epilepsy specialist. Felbamate should be increased slowly. This reduces the risk of side effects. A twice daily administration is possible. If combined with enzyme-inducing antiepileptic drugs such as carbamazepine, phenytoin, or primidone, it may be advisable to administer three dosages daily. This should be determined for individual cases by the epilepsy specialist. The medication is currently available in tablet form of 400 mg and 600 mg as well as in liquid form.

WHAT DO WE TREAT WITH FELBAMATE, AND HOW EFFECTIVE IS IT?

Felbamate is used on patients with partial seizures and grand mal seizures that so far have been resistant to traditional medications, in order to control seizure frequency and severity. In addition, felbamate has been tested and used in the treatment of the Lennox-Gastaut syndrome, an especially severe form of epilepsy requiring a complex treatment pattern. Studies prior to approval (of felbamate) also demonstrated the effectiveness of monotherapy.

Felbamate is only approved as a supplementary or add-on medication with other medications already effective in the treatment of epilepsy. Only after careful consultation between patient and doctor about its potentially severe side effects, compassionate use may be considered.

Before choosing felbamate, it must be shown that a difficult-to-treat form of epilepsy is present. In addition, felbamate can be used in children from the age of 4 with Lennox-Gastaut syndrome as a supplementary medication if all other available and suitable antiepileptic medications have failed to work well. Felbamate monotherapy (used as the only antiepileptic drug) achieved a 50% seizure reduction in 30% of patients with focal seizures. In more than half of all patients with Lennox-Gastaut syndrome, a more than 50% seizure reduction of the significantly impairing seizures with sudden falls could be observed under treatment with felbamate.

WHAT DO YOU NEED TO KNOW ABOUT THE SIDE EFFECTS OF FELBAMATE?

Felbamate has potentially significant and severe side effects that consist of severe blood count deficiencies and/or liver failure. These side effects led to the strict usage requirements. As such, your epilepsy specialist, in cooperation with you, has carefully contemplated the justification for trying out felbamate. Using felbamate *demands that you are thoroughly briefed on its possible side effects,* and that the decision is reached with your family practitioner as well as your epilepsy specialist. If indicators of these severe side effects are present, felbamate treatment must be discontinued immediately. As this medication is relatively new, fewer observations are available, unlike other medications that we have used for years or even decades. Therefore you should take note of any mental or physical side effects that occur during felbamate therapy, and discuss these with your physician, even if they are not mentioned in the product description. (I/FP/E). With the onset of complaints, any course of action should be determined together with your physician. Unskilled handling or discontinuation of the medication on your own can lead to a dangerous increase of seizures. So far, this has only been observed in single cases, where no clear link between the discontinuation of felbamate and an increase in seizures was established. However, we cannot totally exclude this possibility.

Brain and Psyche

Primarily during the initial treatment phase with felbamate, during which the daily dosage is still being stepped up, headaches, dizziness, fatigue, blurry and double vision, and irritability may be noticed. Should the above-mentioned symptoms occur, you should immediately consult your family practitioner, and in severe cases, immediately consult a specialist (FP/E). Quick relief is usually achieved by reducing the dosage, or by a change in schedule of the daily tablet administration. In the event of dizziness, ask a relative or friend to check if your eyes are "shaking." Your doctor calls this "nystagmus" and will gladly explain how to diagnose it. Nystagmus may indicate a slight over-dosage. Frequently, patients who are being treated with antiepileptic medications report impeded physical performance and concentration ability. Research has so far not determined with certainty to what degree felbamate may be responsible for this. Observations to this date suggest that felbamate has no measurable negative impact on intelligence, memory, or attention abilities. It cannot be excluded that in single cases cognitive problems may occur. Should you be concerned, you should immediately consult a specialist (FP/E). A minor adjustment to your therapy may bring relief.

Allergies and Skin

An increase in inflammation in the nose or throat areas, as well as fever, has been documented. Principally, we wish to bring to your attention, once more, that felbamate is a new medication; as such, not all side effects are yet known. Thus you should discuss any unwanted physical or mental changes, even if they have not been stated in the product description, with your consulting physician.

Blood

Severe blood count variations have been documented during felbamate therapy; the most dangerous one is aplastic anemia, which may be a life-threatening condition. It is of significant importance that relevant blood tests are regularly performed in order not to overlook the development of aplastic anemia. Aplastic anemia is a condition in which laboratory results usually indicate its development prior to the appearance of clinical symptoms such as fatigue, feeling of sickness, or lack of energy. If you sense symptoms like this, you should immediately consult your physician, so that your tolerance to felbamate can be determined early (FP/E). Through a quick and timely response (discontinuation of the medication), severe consequences of the side effects are avoided.

Bone

Nothing known.

Gastrointestinal Tract and Internal Organs

Beside aplastic anemia, liver failure is the second life-threatening condition that has been observed with felbamate. Liver tests in the blood are therefore recommended every two weeks. If you sense symptoms such as nausea, vomiting, or a general feeling of sickness, lack of energy, or severe fatigue, then you should immediately consult your physician, so that your tolerance to felbamate can be determined early (FP/E). Through a quick and timely response (discontinuation of the medication), severe consequences of the side effects are avoided.

Apart from the described serious side effects of felbamate, nausea, vomiting, and weight loss may occur. In such cases, consult your doctor first. If the cause for your symptoms cannot be isolated, you may need to see a specialist (S).

Heart

Nothing known.

Interactions with Other Drugs

Numerous interactions may occur with felbamate, both with other antiepileptic drugs and with other drugs in general. Felbamate may increase the serum concentration of phenytoin by up to 60%, of valproate by 20–50%, and of phenobarbital by 25%. Carbamazepine levels drop by 25%, whereas the concentration of carbamazepine epoxide, a metabolite that is sometimes responsible for tolerability problems under carbamazepine, increases. Carbamazepine, phenytoin and phenobarbital decrease the serum concentration of felbamate. The serum concentration of felbamate may rise in combination with valproate.

Contraception, Pregnancy, and Breast Feeding

Felbamate does apparently increase the metabolic activity in the liver. This may impede the contraceptive protection provided by the birth control pill. Epilepsy minimally increased the risk of birth defects even without antiepileptic drugs. There is no evidence that the risk is additionally increased through treatment with felbamate. Animal experiments have not provided indicators of fetal damage due to felbamate. However, the data basis in pregnant women with epilepsy who received felbamate treatment is poor. Thus, felbamate should not be used during pregnancy and breast feeding. Should you discover that you have become pregnant while on felbamate, you should not discontinue the medication on your own accord, as this could lead to an increase in seizures, which may present a greater harm to your baby than felbamate itself. Consult a specialist immediately, and discuss the further course of action.

We have now extensively informed you about the rare but possible side effects of felbamate. You should be aware that your doctor selected this medication as it presents in his or her view the best possible treatment for your epilepsy, while carrying the least amount of side effects.

Success with felbamate therapy is only possible if you take the medication as scheduled. Only in this way will you avoid large fluctuations of the drug in your blood. Once full dosage has been established and maximum blood levels have been reached, the rate of seizures should go down. If the frequency of seizures continues, you should seek the advice of your epilepsy specialist.

Gabapentin | How Does It Work? What Are the Side Effects?

Dear patient,
  Your doctor has prescribed gabapentin for the treatment of your epilepsy.

  Based on years of observations in the management of epilepsies, we want to inform you about the effects and side effects of this medication. In addition to the standard product description that came with your medication, we share with you our expertise in a simple and understandable format. The information here is not intended to replace the product description that came with your medication. However, you should read it thoroughly as well, to filter out important and less important information that pertains to you. This guide provides solid advance information to initiate a detailed consultation with your doctor.

HOW DOES GABAPENTIN WORK? WHAT IS THE CORRECT DOSAGE?

Gabapentin was approved in Canada in 1994. Gabapentin differs biochemically from other antiepileptic drugs. Initially, it was designed to be used to treat spastic paralysis, until its anti-epileptic treatment effects became recognized. Meanwhile, its effectiveness in controlling pain associated with neuropathy has become known. There is evidence that the release of selected neurotransmitters that may trigger or suppress a seizure can be influenced by gabapentin in an unknown way. Most studies reported results with dosages between 600 mg and 1,800 mg. To this date, even larger dosages have provided successful treatment, given that the patient was able to tolerate the medication. In contrast to many other medications, gabapentin dosages can be increased to the maximum within just a few days. The metabolic characteristics of gabapentin suggest administration three times daily. In the event that you have any kidney function problems, you should notify your doctor (FP/S) so that a dosage reduction may be considered. Gabapentin in capsule form is available in dosages of 100 mg, 300 mg, and 400 mg. There are also 600 mg and 800 mg tablets.

WHAT DO WE TREAT WITH GABAPENTIN, AND HOW EFFECTIVE IS IT?

Gabapentin has been prescribed for patients with partial seizures, as well as secondarily generalized tonic-clonic (grand mal) seizures, who have not achieved adequate seizure control. These patients received gabapentin as an add-on medication. All in all, 25% of these patients reported a reduction of seizures by 50%. It must be mentioned that the maximum dosages of 1,800 mg have been administered successfully. New observations suggest that, given an acceptable tolerance, larger dosages up to 3,600 mg appear acceptable. The approval of gabapentin is limited to its use as an add-on drug for patients with focal epilepsies. In addition, gabapentin is approved for the treatment of chronic pain.

WHAT DO YOU NEED TO KNOW ABOUT THE SIDE EFFECTS OF GABAPENTIN?

Side effects requiring a discontinuation of gabapentin therapy are rare. As this medication is still relatively new, fewer observations are available than with medications that have been used for years or decades. We therefore encourage you to report any physical or mental symptoms that you observe while taking gabapentin to your treating doctor (FP/S), even if the observed symptoms were not addressed in the product description. Always obtain professional medical advice whenever you notice a side effect. Incompetent management or discontinuation of the medication without professional consultation can lead to a dangerous increase in seizures. So far, such observations were made in rare cases where a direct relationship between the discontinuation of gabapentin and an increase in seizures could not be shown.

Brain and Psyche

During the initial treatment phase, when the daily dosage is still being stepped up, fatigue, dizziness, and gait unsteadiness may occur (FP/S). Rare observations were slurry speech, tremors, and double vision. In the event of dizziness, ask a relative or friend to check if your eyes are "shaking." Your doctor calls this "nystagmus" and will gladly explain how to diagnose it. Nystagmus may indicate a slight over-dosage. Should the above-mentioned side effects continue, you should not hesitate to contact your doctor immediately or even your specialist (S). These symptoms, as bothersome as they are, usually disappear after the adjustment phase, or after a minor dosage correction. Frequently, patients who are being treated with antiepileptic medication report impeded physical performance and concentration ability. Research has so far not determined with certainty to what degree this medication may be responsible. Observations to this date suggest that gabapentin has no measurable negative impact on intelligence, memory, or attention abilities. However, in some individual cases undesirable symptoms may appear. If you suspect this, consult a specialist. Perhaps relief can be achieved with a minor adjustment in the treatment dosage.

Allergies and Skin

Should you notice changes to your skin, itching, or fever (FP/S), which might be part of an allergic reaction, see your family doctor immediately or go to the nearest emergency department. The clinical trials and the post-marketing experience have not shown an elevated risk for allergies and skin reactions so far.

Blood

In rare cases, a reduction of the white cell counts were observed (FP/S). Therefore, a blood screen should be performed at the beginning of your therapy. If the therapy leads to changes in the lab results, see your specialist immediately.

Bone

Nothing known.

Gastrointestinal Tract and Internal Organs

During the adjustment phase, occasional symptoms of nausea, vomiting, stomach pains, and runny nose were reported. During the course of treatment, an increase of weight was observed in rare cases. See your family doctor (FP) first if you notice these symptoms. If your weight gain is not due to gabapentin, a visit to the specialist may not be necessary.

In rare cases, liver enzymes increase (alkaline phosphatase and gamma-GT). These values initially point only to an increase in liver activity that is required for the metabolism of gabapentin, and can be acceptable at double or even triple values. Should symptoms of fatigue, loss of appetite, or yellow skin tone appear, seek medical assistance immediately. Again, we want to bring to your attention that gabapentin is a new medication, so not all side effects are yet known. You should therefore discuss all unwanted physical and mental symptoms with your physician, including those that are not noted on the product description.

Heart

So far nothing points to serious side effects to the cardiovascular system.

Interactions with Other Drugs

Gabapentin does not undergo clinically relevant interactions with other drugs.

Contraception, Pregnancy, and Breast Feeding

Gabapentin does not increase the metabolic activity in the liver. Therefore hormonal contraception is not affected. Epilepsy minimally increases the risk of birth defects even without antiepileptic drugs. There is no evidence that the risk is increased while being treated with this antiepileptic medication. Animal experiments have not provided indicators of fetal damage due to gabapentin.

Should you discover that you have become pregnant while on gabapentin, you should not discontinue the medication on your own accord, as this could lead to an increase in seizures, which could present a greater harm to your baby than gabapentin itself.

Consult a specialist immediately, and discuss the further course of action.

We have now thoroughly informed you about the rare but possible side effects of gabapentin. You should be aware that your doctor selected this medication because it currently presents the best possible treatment for your epilepsy, with minimal side effects.

Successful gabapentin therapy is only possible if you take the medication as directed. Only in this way will you avoid large fluctuations of the drug in your blood. Once full dosage has been established and maximum blood levels have been reached, the rate of seizures should go down. If this is not the case, seek the advice of your epilepsy specialist immediately.

Lacosamide | How Does It Work? What Are the Side Effects?

Dear patient,

Your doctor has prescribed lacosamide for the treatment of your epilepsy. We want to inform you about the effects and side effects of this medication. In contrast to the standard product description, we will use a simple and understandable format. Lacosamide was approved in both the United States and Europe in 2008, as an add-on treatment for focal seizures, with or without secondary generalization, for epilepsy patients 16 years or older. It is available in Canada through a Special Access Program. Due to the relatively short period since its release, the full scope of clinical effects and side effects will not be known for the next few years. The information here is not intended to replace the product description that came with your medication. Instead, you should read it thoroughly as well, to filter out important and less important information that pertains to you. This guide provides solid advance information to initiate a detailed consultation with your doctor.

HOW DOES LACOSAMIDE WORK? WHAT IS THE CORRECT DOSAGE?

Biochemically, lacosamide is a functionalized amino acid, which means it is the result of a structural change of the amino acid

d-Serine. Lacosamide contains two new and proven active phar-
maceutical ingredients that are not found in other antiepileptic
medications. Lacosamide impacts the sodium channels in that
it gradually strengthens the inactivated (closed) state. This effec-
tively suppresses the typically fast electrical discharge sequences
of neurons, as well as a long continuing excitation of the cells.
Both actions can prevent epileptic seizures. The second, equally
new mechanism observed was the binding to the phosphor protein CRMP-2 (collapsin response mediator protein 2). However,
the actual effect mechanism has yet to be understood.

Lacosamide has been highly effective in various animal tests
in the control of focal onset and generalized seizures, as well as
status epilepticus. Orally administered lacosamide, in tablet form
or syrup, is quickly absorbed by the body, and binds only a small
amount of protein (15%) in the blood. This offers the advantage
that the absorption of lacosamide into the bloodstream is not
impeded if you consume food at the same time. Peak levels of
the medication show up in the blood after about 30 minutes to 4
hours. After about 3 days, the intended drug level (steady state) in
the serum plasma has stabilized. Forty percent of lacosamide is
discharged unchanged, and less than 30% is discharged as inac-
tive waste (O-desmethyl-metabolite). The metabolic activity in the
liver is not significant. The discharge (or in medical terms, elimination) occurs exclusively through the kidneys within a half-life
time of about 13 hours. An increase or decrease of enzyme activity, as has been observed with older medications such as carbamazepine, phenytoin, and phenobarbital is not expected with
lacosamide. Reciprocal effects (interactions) with other medications or substances within your body, such as vitamin D or male
and female sex hormones, will not occur. In case of reduced
kidney function (with the glomerular filtration rate reduced to
below 30 ml/min), especially in older patients, a reduction of the
daily dosage may become necessary. Regularly scheduled serum
plasma screening is not required in this case. Extensive research
data from patients with focal epilepsy are available. In these

controlled studies, lacosamide was administered in dosages ranging between 200 and 600 mg daily, in combination with another
antiepileptic medication. In general, among patients who received
lacosamide, when compared to patients not taking lacosamide,
the study showed significant improvement. Often a dosage of 200
mg proved effective. The recommended daily maximum dosage is
400 mg (200 mg twice daily). When increasing the dosage (from
200 mg to 400 mg), a clear dosage-response relationship can be
shown. The individually required and tolerable lacosamide dosage should be determined together with an epilepsy specialist.
Administration of the medication twice daily is aimed for. During
the first week of treatment, an initial dosage of 50 mg (once in the
morning and once in the evening) is recommended. With good
tolerance, the dosage can be increased during the second week
to twice daily 100 mg. Dependent on further observed tolerance
and effectiveness, the dosage can be increased to 400 mg per day
(200 mg in the morning and evening). With some patients, this
can be done during week 4, while others may require more time.
The individually adapted dosage pattern should be precisely coordinated with the specialist. Lacosamide, for oral administration,
is currently available as a coated tablet (50, 100, 150, 200 mg) and
as syrup (15 mg/ml). In cases where administration in tablet form
or syrup is not possible, intravenous administration (10 mg/ml)
is an option.

WHAT DO WE TREAT WITH LACOSAMIDE, AND HOW EFFECTIVE IS IT?

Lacosamide is currently approved for patients who are 16 years
or older. It is given as an add-on treatment for partial epileptic
seizures and secondarily generalized tonic-clonic (grand mal)
seizures. Lacosamide was tested in three large clinical studies in
Europe, North America, and Australia. These studies focus on

patients with difficult-to-treat epilepsies who failed to respond to several (at least 2 to 3) additional antiepileptic medications. The additional administration of a daily dosage of 400 mg of lacosamide resulted in a reduction of seizures in more than half for 40% of all patients observed. Due to the newness of the medication, only a few long-term study results are available. However, one long-term observation with 370 patients showed that after one year, 77% of the subjects still took lacosamide, which points to a high acceptance and tolerance. Two comparison studies examined lacosamide tablet therapy with lacosamide intravenous therapy. Both studies showed an equal tolerance and an equal treatment effect for either oral (tablets) or intravenous administration. All observations indicated a significant effect of lacosamide in the treatment of epilepsy.

WHAT DO YOU NEED TO KNOW ABOUT THE SIDE EFFECTS OF LACOSAMIDE?

Because lacosamide is a new medication, fewer observations are available as compared to medications that have been used for many years. For this reason, we ask that you report to your doctor any unwanted physical or mental symptoms that you notice after taking lacosamide. Report these even if they are not mentioned in the product description (I/FP/S). Apply this recommendation to any appearance of discomfort you may observe. Incorrect handling or discontinuing the medication on your own increases the risk of an increase in seizures.

Brain and Psyche

During the adjustment phase of the treatment, especially if administered quickly, side effects also observed with several other antiepileptic medications may occur. Dizziness, nausea, coordination difficulties (unsteady gait and inaccurate motor coordination), concentration difficulties, double vision, blurry vision, eye trembling, tremors, headaches, and fatigue may occur. These side effects, observed during the current studies, were clearly dosage-dependent and were mainly observed with dosages above the recommended 400 mg. Usually, these mostly harmless symptoms vanish shortly after treatment has commenced. This may be done by adjusting the dosage. Should these symptoms persist, even after dosage adjustments, it may become necessary to discontinue the medication. Drug tolerance with intravenous administration showed similar results, as did the treatment with tablets. Occasional slight pain at the intravenous site was reported. Psychological symptoms such as depression were only observed in less than 4% of the patients. If you notice a similar side effect, we recommend that you report this immediately to your epilepsy specialist.

Allergies and Skin

Occasional skin irritation (pruritus) was reported during lacosamide therapy. Allergic reactions have only been rarely observed, which again makes it very important that you contact your physician in the event of symptoms affecting the skin or mucus membranes.

The coating of the tablets contains soy lecithin (lipid extracted from soy). Cleaned soy lecithin does not usually trigger allergies, but isolated cases of traces of soy protein may appear. Patients with food allergies to soy products must therefore not take this medication in tablet form. Taking the medication either as syrup or intravenously is not a concern, as these preparations contain no soy lecithin. Lecithins are found in countless food products (pastries, chocolates, marzipan, ice cream, many ready-to-eat meals, and in emulsifying agents). Estimates suggest that 0.1–0.5% of the population has a peanut/soy allergy. If you are aware of any allergy, you must immediately inform your physician prior to taking lacosamide. Again, we want to bring to your attention that lacosamide is a new medication; as such, not all side effects are yet known. You should therefore discuss all unwanted physical and mental symptoms with your physician, including those that are not noted on the product description.

Blood

Nothing known.

Bone

Nothing known.

Gastrointestinal Tract and Internal Organs

Among the side effects with internal organs, complaints to the gastrointestinal system, such as vomiting, flatulence, and constipation, were reported. Changes to body weight observed with other antiepileptic medications have thus far not been observed with lacosamide. So far, no serious side effects on the liver or hematopoietic system have been recorded. Although reports of interferences with internal organs have been made, these did not show a higher frequency of incidents than those observed in the untreated control group (subjects that received placebos). Every newly observed side effect that has not been mentioned here but that shows clear characteristics should be treated as a side effect of lacosamide until proven otherwise. As such, you should immediately consult with your personal physician or epilepsy specialist.

Heart

Depending on the dosage, cardiac examination showed slightly elongated durations of rhythmic cardiac contractions (PR interval). Normally, this is not a health concern. However, if significant cardiac rhythm delays (i.e., AV-block 1st degree) or a tendency to loss of consciousness and bradycardia develop, caution is recommended. In the presence of preexisting cardiac arrhythmias, lacosamide should, in general, not be given.

Interactions with Other Drugs

Lacosamide does not undergo clinically relevant interactions with other drugs.

Contraception, Pregnancy, and Breast Feeding

Lacosamide, unlike older antiepileptic medications, does not accelerate the metabolic rate of the liver. In agreement with a reciprocal effect study, it was shown that the contraceptive protection of the birth control pill, with its hormonal content, was not affected during simultaneous administration of lacosamide. Regarding the risk of bearing a child with deformities or handicaps, human observations are at this point still insufficiently inconclusive to permit a guiding statement. It is also not known if lacosamide transfers into the milk of nursing mothers. Therefore, lacosamide should not be taken during pregnancy or while nursing. Should you become pregnant while on lacosamide therapy, do not discontinue the medication without consulting your doctor. This could lead to an increase in seizures, which could present a greater danger to your child than your lacosamide therapy. Visit your doctor immediately to discuss the best course of action.

We have now thoroughly informed you about the rare but possible side effects of lacosamide. You should be aware that your doctor selected this medication because it currently presents the best possible treatment for your epilepsy, with minimal side effects.

Successful lacosamide therapy is only possible if you take the medication as scheduled. Only in this way will you avoid large fluctuations of the drug in your blood. Once full dosage has been established and maximum blood levels have been reached, the rate of seizures should go down. If this is not the case, you should seek the advice of your epilepsy specialist immediately.

Lamotrigine | How Does It Work? What Are the Side Effects?

Dear patient,

Your doctor has prescribed lamotrigine for the treatment of your epilepsy. Based on years of observations in the management of epilepsies, we want to inform you about the effects and side effects of this medication. In addition to the standard product description that came with your medication, we share with you our expertise in a simple and understandable format. Lamotrigine was approved in 1994 in the United States and in 1995 in Canada after thorough clinical trials. The information here is not intended to replace the product description that came with your medication. Instead, you should read it thoroughly to filter out information that pertains to you. This guide provides solid advance information to initiate a detailed consultation with your doctor.

HOW DOES LAMOTRIGINE WORK?
WHAT IS THE CORRECT DOSAGE?

Lamotrigine reduces the electrical tension of the neural membranes and as such reduces the occurrence of epileptic seizures. Lamotrigine is available in dosage units of 25 mg, 50 mg, and 100 mg, and in dispersible tablets of 2 mg and 5 mg. Generic medications containing lamotrigine are available now and are available in other dosages. The pace at which your doctor will introduce and adjust you to lamotrigine depends on other medication you are currently taking. If you are also taking medications containing valproic acid, then lamotrigine will be discharged from your body slower than usual. This may slow the pace at which your final dosage will be established. In combination with the enzyme inductors (carbamazepine, phenytoin, phenobarbital), which increase the liver metabolic activity, lamotrigine will be excreted faster. It is not a requirement to check plasma levels regularly for the management of this therapy, as is with other antiepileptic drugs, unless side effects occur.

WHAT DO WE TREAT WITH LAMOTRIGINE, AND HOW EFFECTIVE IS IT?

Research has shown that many patients suffering from epilepsy could be sufficiently controlled with lamotrigine after other antiepileptic drugs failed. Twenty-five percent of patients observed showed a reduced frequency of seizures, by more than half. Other patients had a reduction of seizure duration and severity. Initially, lamotrigine was approved as an add-on medication for drug-resistant partial epilepsies. Since then, approval was granted for monotherapy (treatment with a single medication) as well as the initial medication for the treatment of focal and generalized tonic-clonic seizures. The medication has since become one of the most popular antiepileptic drugs to be used in the initial treatment for seizures. In addition, it is recommended as the medication of first choice for partial epilepsies, in most guidelines. Blood serum level screening for therapy management, except with the occurrence of side effects, may not be required as frequently as with other antiepileptic drugs. The liver metabolic activity is not increased at a larger scale, during lamotrigine treatment, as may be the case with numerous other antiepileptic drugs (enzyme inductors).

WHAT DO YOU NEED TO KNOW ABOUT THE SIDE EFFECTS OF LAMOTRIGINE?

Any side effects are cause for you to contact your doctor (FP/S). Being a fairly new medication, all side effects of lamotrigine are not yet known. Thus you should contact your doctor immediately if any unwanted physical or mental impairment is noticed, even if it is not mentioned in the product description.

Brain and Psyche

You may notice fatigue, double vision, headaches, impaired motor coordination, and insomnia (FP/S). A dosage reduction of lamotrigine or other antiepileptic drugs can frequently bring relief. Occasionally, psychological and/or psychiatric side effects have been recorded. Observed were agitation, states of confusion, and restlessness. Insomnia has been reported repeatedly and may lead to significant sleep lack, which per se can lead to worsening of the seizure situation. Some patients with a preexisting handicap showed an increase of aggressive behaviors. Should these symptoms be noticed, consult your doctor on the further course of action.

Allergies and Skin

Occasionally, hair loss was reported. Serious attention must be given the occurrence of redness of the skin, and skin rashes (FP/S). Similar symptoms can also affect the oral/nasal cavity, the eyes, and the genital or perianal regions. A carefully timed drug adjustment period clearly reduces this risk. If you notice a skin rash, immediately discontinue medication and go to the nearest emergency department, and be sure to tell them you are taking lamotrigine and that you wonder if this is a possible drug reaction. As allergic skin rash carries the associated and life-threatening risk of Lyell syndrome or Steven-Johnson syndrome (S/ED!!), so a specialist should be consulted immediately. The same advice applies if fever, influenza-like symptoms, sleepiness, or an increase in the rate of seizures is noticed. Due to the symptoms mentioned above, your doctor will frequently order laboratory tests. Again, we want to bring to your attention that lamotrigine is a new medication; as such, not all side effects are yet known. You should therefore discuss all unwanted physical and mental symptoms with your physician, including those that are not noted on the product description.

Blood

In rare cases, a reduction of the white cell counts was observed (FP/S). Therefore, a blood screen should be performed at the beginning of your therapy. If the therapy leads to changes in the lab results, see your specialist immediately.

Bone

Nothing known.

Gastrointestinal Tract and Internal Organs

Some patients had gastrointestinal complaints while taking lamotrigine (FP/S). The potential risk of liver damage, although very rare, must be factored into the treatment management at the onset of treatment. In combination therapy with other medications, changes to the blood count have been reported. If bleeding from the mucus membrane occurs, you must see your doctor immediately (FP/S). If the rate of seizures (compared to the before-treatment time) increases, a gradual termination of the medication is recommended. The dosage reduction rate must be determined by the doctor.

Heart

Depending on the dosage, cardiac examination showed slightly elongated durations of rhythmic cardiac contractions in a few individuals (PR interval). Clinically relevant problems are not known.

Interactions with Other Drugs

Carbamazepine, phenytoin, phenobarbital, and oxcarbazepine may reduce the serum concentration of lamotrigine by up to 50%. In combination with valproate, the serum concentration may increase to the fourfold level. This is sometimes used to reach a better therapeutic effect. Lamotrigine may increase the concentration of carbamazepine epoxide, a metabolite that is sometimes responsible for tolerability problems with carbamazepine.

Contraception, Pregnancy, and Breast Feeding

Although it has been reported that lamotrigine reduces the blood concentration of the oral contraceptives, it appears to be a less significant issue than is the case with other antiepileptic drugs. It is also known that oral contraceptives, taken concurrently with Lamotrigine, reduce the blood concentrations and efficacy of lamotrigine. These levels increase again if the oral contraceptive is discontinued. You should inform your doctor if you do take oral contraceptives. With the discontinuation of hormonal contraceptives, over-dosage symptoms may occur, such as double vision, dizziness, or seizures (FP/S). Lamotrigine is currently the best-researched medication in terms of pregnancy and breast feeding, as a database with continuously updated and evaluated information is available. This has allowed the manufacturer to mention in the product description that, when used in monotherapy, no known increased risk to the developing fetus exists. However, a recent report suggested that with larger dosages, there is an increased risk of cleft lip.

It must also be considered that the lamotrigine level may drastically drop during pregnancy and then increase after delivery. Seizures during pregnancy, as well as symptoms of over-dosage after giving birth, may be a consequence. Any indication of these problems must be discussed with your doctors immediately (FP/S).

We have now thoroughly informed you about the rare but possible side effects of lamotrigine. You should be aware that your doctor selected this medication because it currently presents the best possible treatment for your epilepsy, with minimal side effects.

Successful lamotrigine therapy is only possible if you take the medication as directed. Only in this way will you avoid large fluctuations of the drug in your blood. Once full dosage has been established and maximum blood levels have been reached, the rate of seizures should go down. If this is not the case, seek the advice of your epilepsy specialist immediately.

Levetiracetam | How Does It Work? What Are the Side Effects?

Dear patient,
Your doctor has prescribed levetiracetam for the treatment of your epilepsy. Based on years of observations in the management of epilepsies, we want to inform you about the effects and side effects of this medication. In addition to the standard product description that came with your medication, we want to share our expertise in a simple and understandable format. Levetiracetam was first approved in the US (1999) and the EU (2000), followed by Canada in 2006 as adjunctive therapy in the treatment of partial onset seizures in adults with epilepsy. Since then, it has received several supplemental indications as monotherapy in focal seizures and adjunctive therapy across both partial and generalised seizures types as well as paediatric use in the US, Canada and the EU. Overall it has established itself as a broadband antiepileptic medication suitable for all age groups. A complete profile of its effectiveness and contra indications cannot be established yet, due to its relative newness. The information here is not intended to replace the product description that came with your medication. Instead, you should read it thoroughly to filter out information that pertains to you. This guide provides solid advance information to initiate a detailed consultation with your doctor.

HOW DOES LEVETIRACETAM WORK? WHAT IS THE CORRECT DOSAGE?

Levetiracetam is derived from the well-known and well-tolerated medication piracetam, a medication that acts on the central nervous system and is particularly used in the treatment of dementias. Most likely, several mechanisms contribute to its effect that differ in function from other antiepileptic medications. Levetiracetam most likely impacts neural channels where calcium and electrolytes determine electrical excitability (action potential). There is also evidence that levetiracetam fosters the suppression of the inhibitory neurotransmitter gamma-aminobutyric acid (GABA). It has since been shown that the medication binds with the protein SV2A in the brain. This is assumed to be the main mechanism. Levetiracetam is quickly absorbed by the body and points to a favorable metabolic profile. Indicators are little protein binding, no liver metabolism, and thus excretion through the kidneys. Extensive studies on treatments with dosages of 1,000 mg to 5,000 mg daily are available. A daily dosage range of 1,000 mg to 3,000 mg is seen as therapeutically effective and is well tolerated. Individually required and tolerable dosages of levetiracetam should be determined by an epilepsy specialist (S). In principle, levetiracetam should be gradually increased to the required target dosage. Generally, good tolerances were observed with an initial dosage of BID (twice) 500 mg during the first week. This can subsequently be increased. Recommended daily dosages range from 1,000 mg to 3,000 mg per day. We recommend that the medication be taken twice daily. Tablets are available in dosage units of 250 mg, 500 mg, and 750 mg. In addition to the tablet, a syrup for oral administration of this medication became available in intravenous solution.

WHAT DO WE TREAT WITH LEVETIRACETAM, AND HOW EFFECTIVE IS IT?

Levetiracetam was initially used to treat patients with partial and secondarily generalized epileptic seizures who did not respond to other antiepileptic medications. Its full efficacy was identified early in typical epileptic-type EEG tracings. Three clinical studies, with more than 1,400 patients suffering from difficult-to-treat epilepsy, showed that levetiracetam (when added to the existing antiepileptic drug) induced in 40% of subjects a reduction of seizure incidence by half. Eight percent of the patients treated with levetiracetam as add-on treatment actually became seizure-free. These early observations convincingly point to the efficacy of levetiracetam. Sufficient data have since indicated that levetiracetam has good effectiveness in monotherapy (used as single antiepileptic medication). For that reason, levetiracetam has been approved for monotherapy treatment of focal epilepsy. There are clear indicators that levetiracetam treats a broad range of epilepsies and is also effective with generalized seizures. Currently, it is also approved, apart from the add-on treatment of partial seizures (with or without spreading to a general seizure), to treat generalized epilepsies for children 4 years and older suffering from juvenile myoclonic epilepsy.

WHAT DO YOU NEED TO KNOW ABOUT THE SIDE EFFECTS OF LEVETIRACETAM?

Since this product has been available for only a few years, not as many observations are at hand as for drugs that have been used for decades. Thus you should report any undesired physical or mental symptoms that you notice while taking levetiracetam. Consult your doctor, even if these symptoms are not mentioned in the product description (FP/S). Unskilled handling or discontinuing the medication on your own accord adds to the risk of an increase in seizures.

Brain and Psyche

If the introduction to the levetiracetam and the adjustment phase are managed at a quick pace, a washed-out feeling, general fatigue, dizziness, unsteadiness, eye tremors (nystagmus), and slurry speech may occur. These mostly harmless symptoms usually go away after the correct dosage is determined, or minor dosage corrections are made. If even after a dosage reduction these symptoms remain, the medication may have to be discontinued. Gradual dosage adjustment reduces the risks of side effects. This requires patience on your part. Don't become discouraged! Impaired physical and intellectual performance also has occasionally been reported. Heightened states of arousal, nervousness leading to insomnia, as well as slight behavioral oddities (especially with mentally handicapped children), have also been observed on occasion. Some patients report significant mood swings. If these symptoms continue or are severe, consult a specialist (FP/S).

Allergies and Skin

In very few instances, allergic reactions and rash have been described. These happened apparently as a result of the coating capsules. Since this coating has been modified, no more cases were observed. Still, should you notice changes to your skin, itching, or fever (FP/S), which might be part of an allergic reaction, see your family doctor immediately or go to the nearest emergency department (ED), although the clinical trials have not shown an elevated risk for allergies and skin reactions so far.

Blood

Nothing known.

Bone

Nothing known.

Gastrointestinal Tract and Internal Organs

Current studies done with levetiracetam show an unexplained but slight increase of infections such as common-cold-type symptoms with runny nose and coughing. These symptoms were always temporary and did not show common diagnostic infection indicators such as blood count fluctuations. Never did these symptoms lead to a discontinuation of the therapy or a major change in therapy management. In case of severe occurrences, you should contact your doctor or specialist (FP/S). Rarely (3%) were significant reductions in blood pigmentation or in red/white cell counts observed. So far, no indicators of serious side effects to the cardiovascular system, the liver, or the blood-building systems have been reported. Allergic reactions, or changes to the skin, have not been reported. Again, we want to bring to your attention that levetiracetam is a new medication; as such, not all side effects are yet known. You should therefore discuss all unwanted physical and mental symptoms with your physician, including those that are not noted on the product description.

Heart

Nothing known.

Interactions with Other Drugs

Levetiracetam does not undergo clinically relevant interactions with other drugs.

Contraception, Pregnancy, and Breast Feeding

Levetiracetam, unlike older antiepileptic medications, does not accelerate the metabolic rate of the liver. Hormonal contraception protection of the contraceptive pill is therefore not affected during concurrent administration of levetiracetam. Epilepsy on its own, even without antiepileptic therapy, marginally raises the risk that a child will be born with a deformity.

Animal studies have so far not indicated fetal damage due to levetiracetam, but as human observations are so far inconclusive, it is recommended that one should not take levetiracetam during pregnancy or when breast feeding. Should you become pregnant during levetiracetam therapy, do not discontinue the medication, as you may risk an increase in seizures, which can be more dangerous to your child than the levetiracetam itself. Instead, consult a specialist immediately and discuss further actions.

We have now thoroughly informed you about the rare but possible side effects of levetiracetam. You should be aware that your doctor selected this medication because it currently presents the best possible treatment for your epilepsy, with minimal side effects.

Successful levetiracetam therapy is only possible if you take the medication as directed. Only in this way will you avoid large fluctuations of the levels of drug in your blood. Once full dosage has been established and proper blood levels have been reached, the rate of seizures should go down. If this is not the case, seek the advice of your epilepsy specialist immediately.

Oxcarbazepine
How Does It Work? What Are the Side Effects?

Dear patient,

Your doctor has prescribed oxcarbazepine for the treatment of your epilepsy. Based on years of observations in the management of epilepsies, we want to inform you about the effects and side effects of this medication. In addition to the standard product description that came with your medication, we share with you our expertise in a simple and understandable format. The information here is not intended to replace the product description that came with your medication. Instead, you should read it thoroughly to filter out information that pertains to you. This guide provides solid advance information to initiate a detailed consultation with your doctor.

HOW DOES OXCARBAZEPINE WORK? WHAT IS THE CORRECT DOSAGE?

Oxcarbazepine was approved in several European countries in early 1990. It finally was approved in the United States in 2000 and in Canada in 2006. Years of research and patient observations in other countries have provided us with good information about its effectiveness and side effects.

Chemically, oxcarbazepine, is a close relative of the well-established antiepileptic medication carbamazepine. It seems to be better tolerated by some patients, with no apparent difference in effectiveness. This is because it metabolizes differently. Oxcarbazepine stabilizes and reduces the electrical tension on the neural membranes and as such reduces the probability of epileptic seizures. Oxcarbazepine is rapidly reduced to the clinically relevant metabolite MHD (10,11-dihydro-10-hydroxy-carbazepine monohydroxy derivative). The individually required dosage of oxcarbazepine differs between patients and depends on the severity of the disease, the weight of the patient, and metabolic issues. By slowly introducing the medication and gradually increasing the dosage to the desired level, one can significantly improve its tolerance. The suitable dosage to treat your individual type of seizures must be determined by your doctor over several appointments. Patience is required, as metabolization takes its time. In view of the way oxcarbazepine is metabolized, a twice-daily administration is recommended. In general, the daily dosage for adults ranges between 1,200 mg and 2,700 mg. The medication is currently available as a tablet in dosage units of 150 mg, 300 mg, and 600 mg and as a suspension (60 mg/ml). An oxcarbazepine sustained-release product (controlled release) is not yet available in Canada, but is available in many other countries (e.g., in Europe). The controlled release causes the level of oxcarbazepine in the bloodstream to remain consistent while MDH, the actual degradation agent and active metabolite, is maintained in high concentrations. This results in better side effect characteristics.

WHAT DO WE TREAT WITH OXCARBAZEPINE, AND HOW EFFECTIVE IS IT?

Oxcarbazepine is used in the treatment of patients with partial and secondarily generalized tonic-clonic seizures (grand mal).

WHAT DO YOU NEED TO KNOW ABOUT THE SIDE EFFECTS OF OXCARBAZEPINE?

Brain and Psyche

During the initial treatment stage, when the daily dosage of oxcarbazepine is gradually increased to the target level, symptoms such as fatigue, dizziness, and an unsteady gait may occur. In the event of dizziness, ask a relative or friend to check if your eyes are "shaking." Your doctor calls this "nystagmus" and will gladly explain how to diagnose it. Nystagmus may indicate a slight over-dosage. If the above symptoms don't go away, contact your family doctor immediately. If the symptoms intensify, contact your epilepsy specialist immediately. Generally, most of these annoying but usually harmless symptoms disappear soon after the adjustment phase, or after a minor dosage correction. Patients who are being treated with antiepileptic drugs occasionally complain about impairment of physical and intellectual properties. Neuropsychological studies have so far not identified a negative impact of oxcarbazepine on intelligence, memory, or attention capacity. However, one cannot fully exclude the possibility of an individual occurrence of such problems. In the event that you suspect that this is so in your case, you should immediately consult a specialist or family physician (FP/S). A small adjustment in your dosage may well bring relief.

Allergies and Skin

Allergic reactions to oxcarbazepine, including suppression and reduction of white blood cells and skin reactions, occur occasionally, as with its close relative carbamazepine.

Should you notice changes to your skin, itching, or fever (FP/S), which might be part of an allergic reaction, see your family doctor immediately or go to the nearest emergency department (ED).

Blood

Occasional blood count variations have been reported during treatment with oxcarbazepine. Worth mentioning is a mostly harmless and temporary reduction of white blood cells (leukocytes). The doctor will monitor your blood count during the therapy, and especially during the adjustment phase (FP/S).

Bone

Although data are missing, it is possible that long-term treatment with oxcarbazepine could have a negative impact on bone density (see below). Therefore the doctor will carefully watch this and decide with you whether the treatment can be continued (FP/S).

Gastrointestinal Tract and Internal Organs

Gastrointestinal side effects are also rare. A slow introduction to the medication may ease or even eliminate these effects.

Liver damage is not expected, even after years of treatment. Increases by two- and threefold in the levels of liver enzyme gamma-GT reading have been observed, but this appears to be no reason for concern—these readings merely indicate the metabolic activity. In very rare cases, an inflammation of the liver has been reported. Should you notice yellow skin color tone, exhaustion, nausea, or loss of appetite, this may be an indicator of liver failure, occurring in very rare cases. *Please seek professional help immediately* (FP/S/ED). Nausea and fatigue may also be due to lowered blood sodium levels, which have been observed particularly in the elderly. Thus, your doctor will regularly monitor the electrolyte levels in your blood. Glaucoma patients should have their intraocular pressure checked on a regular basis.

Heart

In rare cases, in people with a preexisting heart condition, cardiac arrhythmias may occur. Thus be sure to inform your doctor about any preexisting medical conditions (FP/S).

Interaction with Other Drugs

Oxcarbazepine is a mild enzyme inductor. As such, it accelerates the metabolic rate of the liver (thus increasing gamma-GT levels). However, the extent of the enzyme induction is significantly less than that seen with common antiepileptic drugs with similar characteristics. We cannot exclude the possibility that after long-term therapy a shortage of micronutrients (trace elements), hormones, and vitamins may be noticed due to the accelerated degradation. Stay alert for symptoms of these deficiencies, such as reduced bone density, cramps in the calf, and pain in the sole of the foot. In selected cases, a change in medication may be considered. This requires a careful review of the benefit versus risk relationship. It must be noticed that the above-mentioned symptoms may not always stem either partially or fully from the medication (FP/S).

Known interactions concerning antiepileptic drugs are increases of the serum concentrations of phenytoin and phenobarbital. Carbamazepine levels drop, whereas the concentration of carbamazepine epoxide, a metabolite that is sometimes responsible for tolerability problems under carbamazepine, increases. Again, we want to bring to your attention that oxcarbazepine is a new medication; as such, not all side effects are yet known. You should therefore discuss all unwanted physical and mental symptoms with your physician, including those that are not noted on the product description.

Contraception, Pregnancy, and Breast Feeding

Oxcarbazepine does not accelerate the metabolic activity of the liver in the same fashion as other antiepileptic drugs. However, it may still critically affect the contraceptive protection provided by the contraceptive pill. Epilepsy, even if not treated with antiepileptic drugs, carries a slight risk of fetal deformity. This risk is not increased if treated with only one antiepileptic drug. Animal tests have not indicated potential damage to fetal development. However, we always recommend early diagnostics to check on the healthy development of your child. If you become pregnant while already on oxcarbazepine, you should not discontinue the medication on your own accord, as this could lead to an increase in seizures, presenting a greater harm to your baby than oxcarbazepine itself. Consult a specialist immediately, and discuss further course of action.

We have now thoroughly informed you about the rare but possible side effects of oxcarbazepine. You should be aware that your doctor selected this medication because it currently presents the best possible treatment for your epilepsy, with minimal side effects.

Successful oxcarbazepine therapy is only possible if you take the medication as directed. Only in this way will you avoid large fluctuations of the drug in your blood. Once full dosage has been established and optimal blood levels have been reached, the rate of seizures should go down. If this is not the case, seek the advice of your epilepsy specialist immediately.

Perampanel | How Does It Work? What Are the Side Effects?

Dear patient,

Your doctor has prescribed perampanel for the treatment of your epilepsy. We want to inform you about the effects and side effects of this medication. In contrast to the standard product description, we will use a simple and understandable format. Perampanel was approved in Europe and the United States in 2012, as an add-on treatment for focal seizures, with or without secondary generalization, for epilepsy patients 12 years or older. It is licensed in Canada as an add-on treatment for focal seizures in adult patients with epilepsy who are not satisfactorily controlled with conventional therapy. Due to the relatively short period since its release, the full scope of clinical effects and side effects will not be known for the next few years. The information here is not intended to replace the product description that came with your medication. Instead, you should read it thoroughly as well, to filter out important and less important information that pertains to you. This guide provides solid advance information to initiate a detailed consultation with your doctor.

HOW DOES PERAMPANEL WORK?
WHAT IS THE CORRECT DOSAGE?

Perampanel is a once daily, non-competitive AMPA glutamate receptor antagonist, and is the first medication in its class. This effect leads to the reduced effectiveness of glutamate, which is the most important excitatory neurotransmitter in the human brain. Because we think that the excitatory effect of glutamate plays a major role, especially in epilepsy patients, the unique mode of action of perampanel may help in epilepsy patients who were not treated successfully with other antiepileptic drugs with different mechanisms of action.

Perampanel has been highly effective in various animal tests in the control of focal onset and generalized seizures. Orally administered Perampanel is available in tablets with a strength of 2 mg, 4 mg, 6 mg, 8 mg, 10 mg, and 12 mg, respectively. It is quickly absorbed by the body, and binds to a huge amount of protein (95%) in the blood. This means that the amount of the medication that is absorbed by the body from a single tablet changes if the tablet is taken with or without food. However, for the overall amount that is in the blood it is not relevant, because the elimination of the medication is very slow. The elimination half-life is around 105 hours, meaning that after 105 hours about 50% of the drug still remains in the body. After about 14 days of taking perampanel, the intended drug level (steady state) in the bloodstream has stabilized at a steady level. The long elimination half-life offers the opportunity to take perampanel only once daily. In order to reduce typical side effects like dizziness and fatigue, we strongly recommend taking perampanel at bedtime. Most of the drug is metabolized (broken down) in the liver. It has been noted that so-called enzyme-inducing antiepileptic drugs (such as carbamazepine, phenytoin, and some others) may increase the rate of elimination of perampanel considerably. This will need to be considered when adding perampanel to one of those agents. On the other hand, perampanel appears to have only a minor effect on other medications or compounds that are metabolized by the liver. However, we want to repeat that the drug is very new, and experiences with its use in clinical practice are therefore more limited than with any other antiepileptic drug commented on in this book.

Extensive research data from patients with focal epilepsy are available. In these controlled studies, perampanel was administered in dosages ranging between 4 mg and 12 mg daily, in combination with another antiepileptic medications. In general, among patients who received perampanel, when compared to patients not taking perampanel, studies showed significant improvement. The recommended daily maximum dosage is 12 mg (once daily). When increasing the dosage, a clear dosage-response relationship could be shown until 8 mg. In open follow-up studies, it was then shown that in several patients a further increase of the dose may be beneficial. The individually required and tolerable perampanel dosage should be determined together with an epilepsy specialist. Administration of the medication once daily is aimed for. During the first 2 weeks of treatment an initial dosage of 2 mg is recommended. Perampanel should be increased by 2 mg every 2 weeks as needed. In case of the co-administration of an enzyme-inducing antiepileptic drug like carbamazepine or phenytoin, a faster titration may be possible. The epilepsy expert should take responsibility for this decision. The individually adapted dosage pattern should be precisely coordinated with the specialist.

WHAT DO WE TREAT WITH PERAMPANEL, AND HOW EFFECTIVE IS IT?

Perampanel is approved for patients who are 12 years or older. In Canada at this time perampanel is approved for adult patients only. It is given as an add-on treatment for partial epileptic seizures and secondarily generalized tonic-clonic (grand mal) seizures. Perampanel was tested in three large multi-center clinical studies. These studies focus on patients with difficult-to-treat epilepsies who failed to respond to several additional antiepileptic medications. Perampanel was assessed at maintenance dosages of 4 mg, 8mg, and 12 mg, and was compared to add-on placebo (a tablet containing no medication). It was shown that all dosages of perampanel were significantly superior to placebo, so that perampanel was licensed in the doses ranging between 4 mg and 12 mg once daily. More than 90% of patients in the clinical studies were enrolled in an open-label study with perampanel following completion of the study. The rate of patients with a more than 50% seizure reduction increased to and remained at around 50% for the following observation period of one year. Median seizure reduction was also between 40% and more than 50% during this period of open-label treatment with perampanel.

WHAT DO YOU NEED TO KNOW ABOUT THE SIDE EFFECTS OF PERAMPANEL?

Because perampanel is a new medication, fewer observations are available as compared to medications that have been used for many years. For this reason, we ask that you report to your doctor any unwanted physical or mental symptoms that you notice after taking perampanel, even if they are not mentioned in the product description (I/FP/S). Apply this recommendation to any appearance of discomfort you may observe. Incorrect handling or discontinuing the medication on your own increases the risk of an increase in seizures.

Brain and Psyche

During the introduction and dose adjustment phase of the treatment, side effects that are common to many other antiepileptic medications may occur. Dizziness and sleepiness are the leading side effects; others include fatigue, irritability, nausea, and coordination difficulties. Usually these mostly harmless symptoms vanish shortly after treatment has commenced. As mentioned above, these side effects may be minimized by taking the medication at bedtime. Should these symptoms persist, even after dosage adjustments, it may become necessary to discontinue the medication. Serious psychological symptoms, mainly aggression, were observed in less than 3% of patients on perampanel. If you notice a similar side effect, we recommend that you report this immediately to your epilepsy specialist.

Allergies and Skin

Skin reactions have not been reported any more often than with placebo.

Blood

Nothing known.

Bone

Nothing known.

Gastrointestinal Tract and Internal Organs

Weight increase of more than 7% was observed in 14.6% of perampanel-treated patients (2 mg, 12.2%; 4 mg, 14.0%; 8 mg, 15.3%; 12 mg, 15.4 %) versus 7.1% of placebo-treated patients. Over 19 weeks, mean weight gain was greater with perampanel (+1.2 kg) than placebo (+0.4 kg). Other side effects on gastrointestinal tract and internal organs were not observed, but may be still possible. So far, no serious side effects on the liver or hematopoietic system systems have been recorded. Although reports of interferences with internal organs have been made, these did not show a higher frequency of incidents than those observed in the untreated control group (subjects that received placebos). Every newly observed side effect that has not been mentioned here but that shows clear characteristics should be treated as a side effect of perampanel until proven otherwise. As such, you should immediately consult with your personal physician or epilepsy specialist.

Heart

No cardiological side effects or effects on the ECG were observed.

Interactions with Other Drugs

Perampanel is extensively metabolized by the liver. Other antiepileptic drugs that are similarly metabolized may therefore influence the blood level of perampanel. Therefore, under co-administration with carbamazepine, phenytoin, oxcarbazepine, and other so-called enzyme inducers, the serum concentration of perampanel may be lowered so that higher dosages are required to achieve a better antiepileptic effect. Vice versa, perampanel appears to have only a minor effect on the serum concentrations of other antiepileptic drugs.

Contraception, Pregnancy, and Breast Feeding

No effect on levonorgestrel or ethinylestradiol was observed when perampanel was dosed at 4 mg or 8 mg (for 21 days), but perampanel was shown to reduce the total serum concentration of levonorgestrel by approximately 40% when dosed at 12 mg. Therefore we recommend presuming that there may be some interaction, and therefore a reduced effectiveness, of contraceptive protection of the birth control pill when taken with perampanel. Regarding the risk of bearing a child with deformities or handicaps, human observations are at this point still inconclusive to permit a guiding statement. It is also not known if perampanel transfers into the milk of nursing mothers. Therefore, perampanel should not be taken during pregnancy or while nursing. Should you become pregnant while on perampanel therapy, do not discontinue the medication without consulting your doctor. This could lead to an increase in seizures, which could present a greater danger to your child than your perampanel therapy. Visit your doctor immediately to discuss the best course of action.

We have now thoroughly informed you about the rare but possible side effects of perampanel. You should be aware that your doctor selected this medication because it currently presents the best possible treatment for your epilepsy, with minimal side effects.

Successful perampanel therapy is only possible if you take the medication as scheduled. Only in this way will you avoid large fluctuations of the drug in your blood. Once full dosage has been established and maximum blood levels have been reached, the rate of seizures should go down. If this is not the case, seek the advice of your epilepsy specialist immediately.

Phenobarbital/
Primidone | How Does
It Work?
What Are
the Side
Effects?

Dear patient,

Your doctor has prescribed phenobarbital (or the "predrug" primidone, a related drug that breaks down into phenobarbital as part of its metabolization) for the treatment of your epilepsy. Based on years of observation of the management of epilepsies, we want to inform you about the effects and side effects of this medication. In addition to the standard product description that came with your medication, we share with you our expertise in a simple and under-standable format. The information here is not intended to replace the product description that came with your medication. Instead, you should read it thoroughly to filter out information that pertains to you. This guide provides solid advance information to initiate a detailed consultation with your doctor.

HOW DOES PHENOBARBITAL WORK?
WHAT IS THE CORRECT DOSAGE?

The effectiveness of phenobarbital in epilepsy was first discovered in 1912. Since new medications have been introduced, phenobarbital is not the medication of first choice any more. This is mainly due to its side effects, particularly fatigue. However, it may be an effective second choice in cases of difficult-to-treat epilepsies. Phenobarbital stabilizes the electrical activity on the neural membranes. There is also evidence that it increases the seizure-suppressing inhibitory neurotransmitter gamma-aminobutyric acid (GABA) in the brain. Phenobarbital metabolizes slowly. This means that the time needed to reach the desired stable blood levels may be 3 to 4 weeks. Only then can its effect be determined. Of note is that withdrawal seizures may occur if the medication is suddenly discontinued.

Primidone was introduced as an antiepileptic drug in 1952. Seventy percent is converted to phenobarbital in the body. Whether primidone in itself contains a seizure-suppressing agent, as does phenobarbital, is not certain, but probable. Primidone will be metabolized to phenobarbital, which is antiepileptic.

The following applies to adult patients: phenobarbital is generally administered in daily dosages of 100 to 300 mg (= 1–3 tablets @ 100 mg each). The daily dosage of primidone at the median is between 0.75 g and 1.5 g. A daily dosage of 100 mg of primidone would represent the equivalent dosage of 60 mg of phenobarbital. Phenobarbital tablets are available in dosage units of 15 mg, 30 mg, 60 mg, and 100 mg; primidone is available in 250 mg tablets.

WHAT DO WE TREAT WITH PHENOBARBITAL, AND HOW EFFECTIVE IS IT?

You are receiving a strong seizure-suppressing medication to treat focal and generalized tonic-clonic seizures (grand mal). Awakening grand mal seizures seem to respond very well to phenobarbital. Seizure freedom can be achieved in 60% of those treated. Fifty percent of those treated for complex partial seizures have become seizure free when treated in combination therapy with other medications. It has very good efficacy data in a wide range of other generalized seizure types; thus, it achieves complete seizure control in 80% of all cases with juvenile myoclonic seizures. Compared with carbamazepine and phenytoin, phenobarbital is better tolerated by the gastrointestinal tract. It also causes fewer allergies or changes in the blood profile.

WHAT DO YOU NEED TO KNOW ABOUT THE SIDE EFFECTS OF PHENOBARBITAL?

Brain and Psyche

Current data indicate that a long-term therapy with phenobarbital may impact cognitive functions in growing children. Some children show behavioral symptoms of fatigue, restlessness, and aggressive tempers.

Phenobarbital treatment of adults often causes tiredness and fatigue. Cautious dosage management during the adjustment phase may lessen this side effect, and fatigue may eventually diminish. Depression and impaired cognitive performance are occasionally observed with phenobarbital therapy. Only with a small group of patients has it become necessary to discontinue the medication because of these side effects.

Allergies and Skin

Major allergic reactions are rare, but when starting treatment, skin reactions may occur and even need emergency consultation.

After initiation of the therapy (7th–10th day), rashes, similar in appearance to measles, may occur (FP/S). These are generally harmless and disappear when the dosage is reduced. Discontinuation of the medication is rarely required. The transition to more severe allergic reaction is indicated by the appearance of blisters on the skin and fever. If this happens, you must immediately consult your doctor (FP/S/ED). Another very rare symptom is the development of acne.

Blood

Side effects impacting blood-producing bone marrow functions (reduction of white and red cells) are rare and controllable if carefully monitored. One form of anemia, "megaloblastic anemia," is easily treated with folic acid or vitamin B12. Reducing the dosages or withdrawal will lead to a recovery of the reduction of white and red cells. Close contact with your physician is crucial. Coagulation problems with newborns as a result of vitamin K deficiency are managed with vitamin K administration (FP/S).

Bone

Occasional decalcification has been observed during long-term therapy with phenobarbital, especially in patients limited in their mobility during low daylight seasons. In severe cases (i.e., aching bones) treatment with vitamin D is required (FP/S). Phenobarbital belongs to the group of enzyme inductors, which means that it accelerates liver metabolism and can lead to increase in the liver enzyme gamma-GT. In long-term therapy this may lead to a deficiency of trace elements, hormones, or vitamins due to their accelerated degradation. Therefore it becomes necessary that you look for indicators of these deficiencies with symptoms such as reduced bone mineral density, nightly calf cramps, and aching foot soles. The accelerated degradation of other medications will subsequently reduce their efficacy, which may require a change in the medication. On an individual basis, this will occasionally require a careful analysis of risk and benefits. It must always be considered that these symptoms may not be entirely due to this medication. Further rare side effects include stiff shoulders, thickening of the connective tissue, especially in the palm of the hand, swelling of the legs, thirst, and frequent passing of urine.

Gastrointestinal Tract and Internal Organs

Phenobarbital is a strong enzyme inductor. This means that it accelerates the metabolic rate of the liver. Levels of the enzyme gamma-GT can increase two- to sixfold in about 90% of those treated with this medication. By this mechanism, phenobarbital frequently inactivates sexual hormones and vitamin D. This results in erectile dysfunction in men and menstrual irregularities in women, as well as osteoporosis. Medication you are taking concurrently, including antiepileptic drugs, may be weakened significantly. However, even after taking this medication for decades, no long-term changes to the liver cells have been observed, while all other liver values remained in the normal range. You should therefore avoid any additional burden on the liver, as for example due to the consumption of alcoholic beverages.

A small reduction of thyroid hormones may be the result of phenobarbital therapy. However, treatment with thyroid hormones is only required if symptoms of a hypothyroidism (underproduction of thyroid hormone) occur.

Heart

No common side effects have to be considered.

Interaction with Other Drugs

Phenobarbital is an enzyme inducer, which accelerates the metabolic rate of the liver (resulting in the above described increase in gamma-GT). Therefore the serum levels of other antiepileptic drugs, but also of other drugs that are given because of other indications beyond epilepsy, may fall. This can be clinically relevant if the effects of these drugs are not as expected. A dose adaptation may be necessary (FP/S).

Contraception, Pregnancy, and Breast Feeding

Phenobarbital reduces the efficacy of the contraceptive pill as it increases the liver's metabolic rate. The reliability of medicated contraception is thus diminished. Discuss other methods of birth control with your physician and/or your gynecologist. Phenobarbital seems not to increase the risk of fetal deformities significantly as long as this is the only medication taken (monotherapy). Primidone carries, compared to phenobarbital, a much higher risk of fetal deformity (S). It is well-known that occasional newborns will have vitamin K deficiency. Administering vitamin K even prior to giving birth is a common way to prevent this, and helps reduce the risk of bleeding. Less than 50% of phenobarbital is carried into mother's breast milk. Some observations have suggested an impact on the cardiovascular functions of newborns, but this finding was not consistent in other studies. All studies point to additional fatigue and weaker sucking by the baby as a result of this medication. In such cases you must discontinue breast feeding—of course gradually, in order to avoid withdrawal symptoms.

We have now thoroughly informed you about the rare but possible side effects of phenobarbital. You should be aware that your doctor selected this medication because it currently presents the best possible treatment for your epilepsy, with minimal side effects.

Successful phenobarbital therapy is only possible if you take the medication as directed. Only in this way will you avoid large fluctuations of the drug in your blood. Once full dosage has been established and optimal blood levels have been reached, the rate of seizures should go down. If this is not the case, seek the advice of your epilepsy specialist immediately.

Phenytoin | How Does It Work? What Are the Side Effects?

Dear patient,
Your doctor has prescribed phenytoin for you to treat your epilepsy. Based on years of observations in the management of epilepsies, we want to inform you about the effects and side effects of this medication. In addition to the standard product description that came with your medication, we share with you our expertise in a simple and understandable format. The information here is not intended to replace the product description that came with your medication. Instead, you should read it thoroughly to filter out information that pertains to you. This guide provides solid advance information to initiate a detailed consultation with your doctor.

HOW DOES PHENYTOIN WORK?
WHAT IS THE CORRECT DOSAGE?

The American researchers H. Houston Merritt and Tracy Putnam originally discovered the seizure-suppressing properties of phenytoin in 1938. Phenytoin was the result of further development work with a chemically related barbiturate, which at the time was being used to treat epilepsy. In contrast to its predecessor, phenytoin has less sedative effect and provides better control over typically challenging complex-partial ("psychomotor") seizures. This medication has been available worldwide for many decades. Its active agents primarily stabilize (settle) excited neural membranes and also suppress the spreading of a seizure. Phenytoin is slowly absorbed in the gastrointestinal tract and metabolized in the liver. A high percentage binds with proteins in the blood. The recommended therapeutic dosage is 5 mg/kg body weight. The daily dosage for adults is between 250 mg and 400 mg. Phenytoin comes in capsules of 30 mg and 100 mg, tablet of 50 mg, and suspension of 30 mg/5 ml or 125 mg/5 ml. Due to a slow metabolic rate, the medication can be taken once per day (i.e., 3 tablets in the evening). Even slightly elevated dosages can quickly lead to an overdose. Thus, under no circumstances should you change your dosage without consulting your doctor. If the oral dosage is considered insufficient, then the medication can also be given intravenously (an added benefit over many other antiepileptic medications).

Interactions with other medications are frequent. For that reason you must inform your doctor about all other medications you are currently taking. Here are some illustrative examples. Aspirin® (acetylsalicylic acid), for example, frequently administered to control a fever or in stroke prophylaxis, can increase the strength of phenytoin and lead to an overdose. On the other hand, phenytoin weakens the effectiveness of carbamazepine, corticosteroids, and hormonal preparations (FP/S). Phenytoin levels are often increased if concurrently administrated with blood thinners such as Warfarin®.

WHAT DO WE TREAT WITH PHENYTOIN, AND HOW EFFECTIVE IS IT?

Phenytoin is one of the best-researched antiepileptic medications, based on a wealth of observations. It has proven highly effective against grand mal seizures (at any the time of day) as well as partial seizures with or without loss of consciousness. Depending on the type of seizure, up to 70% of patients showed significant improvement (reduction of or even suppression of seizures) after the initial adjustment phase. Phenytoin has also been effective in emergency treatment situations such as status epilepticus as it can also be administered intravenously.

WHAT DO YOU NEED TO KNOW ABOUT THE SIDE EFFECTS OF PHENYTOIN?

With every desired benefit a medication provides, some side effects are present. Only common and clinically relevant side effects are discussed here. Thus, if you experience what you suspect to be a side effect that has not been mentioned here, you should communicate this to your doctor.

Brain and Psyche

Most side effects are dosage-dependent and are limited to the adjustment phase. Using an A.M. (morning) dosage reduction, side effects such as double vision, blurry vision, unsteady balance, slurry speech, dizziness, and nausea may be eliminated (FP/S). In rare cases, side effects have forced a discontinuation of the medication. In the event of dizziness, ask a relative or friend to check if your eyes are "shaking." Your doctor calls this "nystagmus" and will gladly explain how to diagnose it. Nystagmus may indicate a slight over-dosage. If the above symptoms don't go away, contact your family doctor immediately. If the symptoms intensify, contact your epilepsy specialist immediately. These symptoms often disappear after a small dosage reduction, or by distributing the administration of dosage over the day. Due to its unique metabolic course, a risk of over-dosage exists even during long-term therapy. Intellectual and memory processes may become slightly affected during phenytoin therapy. Occasionally peripheral nerve disorders have been reported. These are noticed as a pins-and-needles sensation or cramps in the calf.

Allergies and Skin

Allergy-type skin rashes have occasionally occurred, especially if the dosage was quickly increased. If you notice a blistery type skin condition, feel generally ill, or notice a swelling of a lymph gland, you need to seek medical help immediately. *Go directly to the nearest emergency department.* Rare skin symptoms include an increase in pigmentation and hair growth (FP/S). Gums can also swell (FP/S), especially in children during the early stage of the therapy.

Blood

Temporary reduction of white cells may occur. Very rarely are other blood cells affected. In all cases, blood counts should be monitored during the adjustment phase.

Bone

Occasionally phenytoin reduces vitamin D levels (especially in children, which makes a sore throat more likely). Much rarer is underperformance of the thyroid gland. Regular blood tests allow early diagnosis of megaloblastic anemia. Phenytoin belongs to the enzyme inductors, which accelerate the liver's metabolic activity and may lead to increase of liver enzyme gamma-GT). During long-term therapy this may lead to a shortage of micronutrients (trace elements), hormones, or vitamins, caused by the acceler-ated degradation. Therefore it becomes necessary that you pay attention to indicators of these deficiencies, such as reduced bone mineral density, nightly calf cramps, and aching foot soles. The accelerated degradation of other medications will subsequently reduce their efficacy, which may require you to consider switch-ing the medication (FP/S). This will require careful consideration of risk and benefits and the understanding that not all of these symptoms are possibly a consequence of this medication.

Gastrointestinal Tract and Internal Organs

Phenytoin is a strong enzyme inductor. This means that it accelerates the metabolic rate of the liver. Levels of liver enzymes (gamma-GT) can increase by two- to sixfold in about 90% of those treated with this medication. By this mechanism, phenytoin frequently reduces levels of sexual hormones and vitamin D, causing erectile dysfunction in men and menstrual irregularities in women, as well as osteoporosis. The effects of medication taken concurrently, including antiepileptic drugs, may be weakened significantly. However, even after taking this medication for decades, no long-term changes to the liver cells have been observed, while all other liver values remained in the normal range. You should therefore avoid any additional burden on the liver, as for example with the consumption of alcoholic beverages.

Heart

Phenytoin has an impact on heart conduction, for which reason it was once used as a drug for patients with arrhythmias. Usually oral medication with phenytoin causes no side effects, but, in emergencies and during an intravenous application, it is mandatory to infuse the drug slowly in order to avoid any adverse reactions.

Interaction with Other Drugs

Phenytoin is an enzyme inducer and accelerates the metabolic rate of the liver (resulting in the above described increase in gamma-GT). Therefore the serum levels of other antiepileptic drugs (and also of other drugs given for indications other than epilepsy) may fall. This can be clinically relevant if the effects of these drugs are not as expected. A dose adaptation may be necessary (FP/S), but adjusting the dose of any medication should only be done in collaboration with your doctor.

Contraception, Pregnancy, and Breast Feeding

Phenytoin reduces the efficacy of the contraceptive pill as it increases the liver metabolic rate. The reliability of medicated contraception is thus diminished. The risk of fetal deformity during phenytoin therapy can be expected to double. However, 98–99% of all treated mothers give birth to healthy children. It must also be noted that frequent epileptic seizures most likely present a greater danger to the unborn than the medication itself. Never reduce or discontinue phenytoin therapy on your own. It must be managed by your physician to protect your baby. Breast feeding is recommended, although a small amount of phenytoin is carried into the breast milk. As a result of this, the development of the child and phenytoine blood serum levels should be monitored regularly (FP/S).

We have now thoroughly informed you about the rare but possible side effects of phenytoin. You should be aware that your doctor selected this medication because it currently presents the best possible treatment for your epilepsy, with minimal side effects.

Successful phenytoin therapy is only possible if you take the medication as directed. Only in this way will you avoid large fluctuations of the drug in your blood. Once full dosage has been established and optimal blood levels have been reached, the rate of seizures should go down. If this is not the case, seek the advice of your epilepsy specialist immediately.

Pregabalin | How Does It Work? What Are the Side Effects?

Dear patient,

Your doctor has prescribed pregabalin for the treatment of your epilepsy. Based on years of observations in the management of epilepsies in many countries around the world, we want to inform you about the effects and side effects of this medication. In addition to the standard product description that came with your medication, we share with you our expertise in a simple and understandable format. The information here is not intended to replace the product description that came with your medication. Instead, you should read it thoroughly to filter out information that pertains to you. This guide provides solid advance information allowing you to initiate a detailed discussion with your doctor. Pregabalin is available in most countries. However, it is currently not officially licensed in Canada for the treatment of epilepsy (only for pain). Pregabalin was approved for epilepsy treatment in the European Market and in the United States in 2004. Pregabalin is used to treat partial seizures and secondarily generalized tonic-clonic seizures in patients 18 years or older. Pregabalin is also prescribed in the United States and the European Union to treat neuropathic pains in diabetics, as well as for the treatment of post-herpetic neuralgia. Due to the relatively short period since its release, the full scope of clinical effects and side effects will not be known for the next few years.

HOW DOES PREGABALIN WORK?
WHAT IS THE CORRECT DOSAGE?

Pregabalin most likely contains several active agents. The intent during development was to modulate the molecule of the well-understood neurotransmitter GABA (gamma-butyric acid). However, its anti-seizure efficacy is believed not to be directly linked to GABA. Its assumed main mechanism is the reduction of the intracellular calcium flow in hyper-excitable neurons. Pregabalin binds to a special neural receptor before the synapse. This effect suppresses the release of an excitatory neurotransmitter called glutamate. Pregabalin is quickly and completely absorbed by the body and does not bind to proteins. It is excreted nearly unchanged through the kidneys, with half value being excreted within 6 to 7 hours.

Pregabalin is not metabolized in the liver, as is the case with several, primarily older, antiepileptic drugs such as carbamazepine, phenytoin, and phenobarbital. Liver enzyme induction is minimal, so unfavorable reactions in the body relating to bone and sex hormones are not expected. In addition, pregabalin does not inhibit the effect of the birth control pill. Pregabalin is not metabolized in the liver, as is the case with several older, antiepileptic drugs such as carbamazepine, phenytoin, and phenobarbital. Liver enzyme induction is minimal, so unfavorable reactions in the body relating to bone and sex hormone metabolism and interactions with other medications are not to be expected. Reduced renal function requires a dosage reduction. This must be closely observed, especially with older patients. After 1 to 2 days, steady-state equilibrium is established. The first antiepileptic effect can be expected within 1 week. The need for blood profile monitoring is currently being evaluated.

There are several studies focusing on combination therapy with pregabalin using a daily dosage range of 300 mg to 600 mg. These dosages were shown to be tolerable and effective. A clear dosage-effect relationship can be shown by increasing the dosage from 300 mg to 600 mg. The initially required and tolerable dosage (target dosage) should be determined together with your epilepsy specialist (FP/S). During the first week of treatment, a dosage of 2 x 75 mg twice daily is recommended. If good tolerance is indicated, the dosage can be increased to 2 x 150 mg beginning in the second week. Depending on further tolerance indications, as well as its medical efficacy, the daily dosage may be increased to 600 mg (2 x 300 mg). Some patients can tolerate this already in the third week, whereas others may require more time. The specialist will help you to find the individually tailored final dosage (S).

The medication is currently available in tablet form in dosage units of 75 mg, 150 mg, and 300 mg. Pregabalin is currently used only as an add-on treatment for focal seizures (with or without the tendency to spread to more generalized seizures). This medication is not approved for monotherapy in many countries and is only available in Canada via special access programs.

WHAT DO WE TREAT WITH PREGABALIN, AND HOW EFFECTIVE IS IT?

Pregabalin is currently approved in many countries for the treatment of adults with focal as well as large epileptic seizures, when conventional drugs did not bring sufficient relief. Its effect is limited to the treatment of partial (simple, complex, and secondarily generalized) seizures. Several comprehensive studies focused on this group of patients who had already been treated unsuccessfully with four to six antiepileptic drugs showed a reduction of up to 40% of seizures affected by the introduction of pregabalin to

the treatment regimen. These observations proved the strong efficacy of pregabalin in the treatment of epilepsy. It is approved for
the treatment of neuropathies in some countries. In some countries it is also approved to treat anxieties and to regulate sleep.

WHAT DO YOU NEED TO KNOW ABOUT THE SIDE EFFECTS OF PREGABALIN?

Since this product has been available for only a few years, not as
many observations are at hand as for drugs that have been used
for decades. Thus you should report to your doctor any undesired
physical or mental symptoms that you notice while taking pregabalin, even if these are not mentioned in the product description
(FP/S). This applies to any related complaints. Unskilled handling
or discontinuing the medication on your own accord adds the risk
of an increase in seizures.

Brain and Psyche

The most frequent of the unwanted side effects were observed
in the area of brain function and psyche, where most of these
were only temporary. During the adjustment phase, especially
if increased quickly, symptoms such as general fatigue, apathy,
unsteady gate, tremors, inaccurate motor movements, double
or blurred vision, speech impairment, and dizziness may occur.
Normally these symptoms disappear a short time after the
adjustment phase has been completed, or after a minor dosage
correction. Should any of these symptoms, even after a dosage
correction, remain or be sufficiently severe, the medication may
need to be discontinued. Memory and concentration problems
have been reported. Furthermore, there are reports of mood
swings, depression, euphoria, and confusion, as well as either
increased or diminished sexual drive (libido) and restlessness.

There are rare reports of illusions and hallucinations. If you notice any of these side effects, then you should quickly contact your epilepsy specialist (FP/S). Pregabalin is also known to relieve anxiety symptoms.

Allergies and Skin

Reports of allergic reactions and skin changes are rare, but pregabalin is not necessarily the cause. However, it is important that if any changes to skin or mucous membranes appear, you should contact your family physician, and if more questions remain unanswered, you should consult a specialist (FP/S).

Blood

Not known.

Bone

Not known.

Gastrointestinal Symptoms and Internal Organs

A frequent side effect reported in the approval studies was weight gain, partially tied to a swelling of the legs (edema). These may also appear separate from each other. A weight gain of about 7% was observed in every tenth patient. Less than 4% of the patients observed increased their weight by a quarter of their original weight. The mechanism of this weight gain is currently being studied, but conclusive results are not yet available, though increased appetite during pregabalin therapy may be a factor. Reported symptoms from the gastrointestinal region were flatulence, constipation, vomiting, and dry mouth. So far there are no reports of side effects on the liver. Occasionally men have reported erectile dysfunction: Please discuss this possible side effect openly with your physician if you experience such symptoms. Again, we want to bring to your attention that pregabalin is a new medication; as such, not all side effects are yet known. You should therefore discuss all unwanted physical and mental symptoms with your physician, including those that are not noted on the product description.

Heart

Very rare are an increase in cardiac rate (tachycardia), impeded cardiac performance, excessive perspiration, or muscle stiffness. Every observed symptom that is not listed here but is lasting and severe must be considered to be a side effect of pregabalin, until proven otherwise, and is a reason for you to see your family practitioner or your specialist.

Interactions with Other Drugs

Pregabalin does not undergo clinically relevant interactions with other drugs.

Contraception, Pregnancy, and Breast Feeding

Pregabalin, unlike older antiepileptic medications, does not accelerate the metabolic rate of the liver. In agreement with a reciprocal effect study, it was shown that the hormonal content and contraceptive protection of the birth control pill were not affected during concurrent administration of pregabalin. Epilepsy minimally increases the risk of birth defects even if the mother is not taking antiepileptic drugs, but the risk is not increased under treatment with this medication.

Pregabalin, when used to treat epilepsy, is administered as an adjunct medication only. Research on mice did not point to any subsequent birth defects. Research on rats, done with double the maximum dosage, showed only occasional impact on development as well as a reduction in fertility. Should you discover that you have become pregnant while on pregabalin treatment, you should not discontinue the medication on your own accord, as this could lead to an increase in seizures, which could present a greater danger to your baby than pregabalin itself. Instead, consult a specialist immediately, and discuss the further course of action.

We have now thoroughly informed you about the rare but possible side effects of pregabalin. You should be aware that your doctor selected this medication because it currently presents the best possible treatment for your epilepsy, with minimal side effects.

Successful pregabalin therapy is only possible if you take the medication as directed. Only in this way will you avoid large fluctuations of the drug in your blood. Once full dosage has been established and optimal blood levels have been reached, the rate of seizures should go down. If this is not the case, seek the advice of your epilepsy specialist immediately.

Retigabine | How Does It Work? What Are the Side Effects?

Dear patient,
Your doctor has prescribed retigabine for the treatment of your epilepsy. We want to inform you about the effects and side effects of this medication. Based on years of observations in the management of epilepsies in many countries around the world, we want to inform you about the effects and side effects of this medication. In addition to the standard product description that came with your medication, we share with you our expertise in a simple and understandable format. Retigabine was approved in both the United States and Europe for introduction to the market in 2011, as an add-on treatment for epilepsy patients 16 years or older, with focal seizures with or without secondary generalization. Due to the relatively short period since the finalization of the clinical trials conducted with retigabine, the full scope of clinical effects and side effects will not be known for the next few years. The information here is not intended to replace the product description that came with your medication. Instead, you should read it thoroughly as well, to filter out important and less important information that pertains to you. This guide provides solid advance information to initiate a detailed consultation with your doctor.

HOW DOES RETIGABINE WORK?
WHAT IS THE CORRECT DOSAGE?

Biochemically, retigabine is an amino ester that is structurally not related to other antiepileptic compounds. Retigabine has a new mode of action, that is, the activation and opening of certain neuronal potassium channels. In addition, it increases the efficacy of the inhibitory neurotransmitter gamma-aminobutyric acid (GABA) in the brain. As a secondary mechanism, it also blocks the synthesis of neuroactive amino acids and GABA itself.

Retigabine has been highly effective in various animal tests in the control of focal onset and generalized seizures, as well as status epilepticus. Orally administered retigabine is quickly absorbed by the body at a rate of 60%, which is not influenced by food. Maximum blood concentrations are measured 1.5 hours after a single oral dose. Elimination half-life is 8 hours, so it is advisable to take retigabine three times per day. Retigabine and its main metabolites are predominantly excreted via the kidney.

Extensive research data from patients with focal epilepsy are available. In these controlled studies, retigabine was administered in dosages ranging between 600 mg and 1,200 mg daily, in combination with another antiepileptic medication. In general, significant improvements were shown with retigabine compared to placebo. A dose of 600 mg proved effective for many patients in the study. The recommended daily maximum dosage will be 1,200 mg. When increasing the dosage, a clear dosage-response relationship can be shown. The individually required and tolerable retigabine dosage should be determined with the epilepsy specialist. Administration of the medication three times daily is aimed for. During the first week of treatment an initial dosage of 300 mg (100 mg three times per day) is recommended. With good tolerance, the dosage can be increased during the second week by 150 mg (50 mg three times per day). Dependent on further observed tolerance and effectiveness, the dosage can be increased to 1,200 mg/day (400 mg three times a day). With some patients this can be done within a relatively short period of time, while others may require more time. The individually adapted dosage pattern should be precisely coordinated with the specialist.

WHAT DO WE TREAT WITH RETIGABINE, AND HOW EFFECTIVE IS IT?

Retigabine is approved for patients who are 16 years or older. It is given as an add-on treatment for focal epileptic seizures and focal seizures with secondarily generalized tonic-clonic (grand mal) seizures. Retigabine was tested in three large clinical studies in Europe, North America, and Australia. These studies focused on patients with difficult-to-treat epilepsies, who failed to respond to one to three additional antiepileptic drugs. The additional administration of a daily dosage of 600 mg of retigabine resulted in a reduction of seizures by more than half in 23% to 39% of all of the patients observed. With 900 mg this was achieved in 32% to 47% of patients; and with 1,200 mg in 33% to 55%. Due to the newness of the medication only a few long-term study results are available.

WHAT DO YOU NEED TO KNOW ABOUT THE SIDE EFFECTS OF RETIGABINE?

Because this is a new medication, fewer observations are available as compared to medications that have been used for many years. For this reason, we ask that you to report to your doctor *any* unwanted physical or mental symptoms that you notice after taking retigabine, even if they are not mentioned in the product description (I/FP/S). Apply this recommendation to any appearance of discomfort you may observe. Incorrect handling or discontinuing the medication on your own increases the risk of an increase in seizures.

Brain and Psyche

During the adjustment phase of the treatment, especially if administered quickly, side effects also observed with several other antiepileptic medications may occur. The higher the dosage, the higher the probability of such side effects. The leading adverse events are somnolence, dizziness, confusion, speech disorder, vertigo, tremor, amnesia, abnormal thinking, and abnormal gait.

Usually these mostly harmless symptoms vanish shortly after treatment has commenced, especially after adjusting the dosage. Should these symptoms persist, even after dosage adjustments, it may become necessary to discontinue the medication.

Allergies and Skin

These are not yet known. However, it is important that if any symptoms appear on skin or mucous membranes, you contact your family physician, and if more questions remain unanswered, that you consult the specialist (FP/S).

Blood

Not known.

Bone

Not known.

Gastrointestinal Tract and Internal Organs

Among the side effects involving internal organs, complaints to the gastrointestinal system, such as nausea and bladder dysfunction (retention, painful urination, or delayed urination), have been reported. However, long-term studies did not show any evidence for an increase of urinary retention. Changes to body weight observed with other antiepileptic medications, have not been observed with retigabine thus far, and no serious side effects to the liver or hematopoietic systems have been recorded. Although reports of interferences with internal organs have been made, these did not show a higher frequency of incidents than those observed in the untreated control group (subjects that received placebos). Every newly observed side effect that has not been mentioned here but that shows clear characteristics should be treated as a side effect of retigabine until proven otherwise, and if they occur you should immediately consult with your personal physician or epilepsy specialist.

Heart

Depending on the dosage, cardiac examination (EKG) may show slightly elongated durations of rhythmic cardiac contractions (QT interval). Normally this is not a health concern.

Interactions with Other Drugs

Few interactions have been described so far. Retigabine decreases the serum concentration of lamotrigine slightly. Whereas lamotrigine increases the serum concentration of retigabine, carbamazepine and phenytoin decrease it. Clinically relevant interactions with phenobarbital, valproate, and topiramate were not found.

Contraception, Pregnancy, and Breast Feeding

Retigabine, unlike older antiepileptic medications, does not accelerate the metabolic rate of the liver. In agreement with a reciprocal effect study, it was shown that the hormonal content and contraceptive protection of the birth control pill were not affected during simultaneous administration of retigabine. Regarding the risk of bearing a child with deformities or handicaps, human observations are at this point still insufficiently inconclusive to permit a guiding statement. It is also not known if retigabine transfers into the milk of nursing mothers. Therefore, retigabine should not be taken during pregnancy or while nursing. Should you become pregnant while on retigabine therapy, do not discontinue the medication without consulting your doctor. This could lead to an increase of seizures, which could present a greater danger to your child than your retigabine therapy. Visit your doctor immediately to discuss the best course of action.

We have now thoroughly informed you about the rare but possible side effects of retigabine. You should be aware that your doctor selected this medication because it currently presents the best possible treatment for your epilepsy, with minimal side effects.

Successful retigabine therapy is only possible if you take the medication as scheduled. Only in this way will you avoid large fluctuations of the drug in your blood. Once full dosage has been established and optimal blood levels have been reached, the rate of seizures should go down. If this is not the case, seek the advice of your epilepsy specialist immediately.

Rufinamide | How Does It Work? What Are the Side Effects?

Dear patient,

Your doctor has prescribed rufinamide for the treatment of your epilepsy. Based on years of observations in the management of epilepsies in many countries around the world, we want to inform you about the effects and side effects of this medication. In addition to the standard product description that came with your medication, we share with you our expertise in a simple and understandable format. The information here is not intended to replace the product description that came with your medication. Instead, you should read it thoroughly to filter out information that pertains to you. This guide provides solid advance information to initiate a detailed consultation with your doctor. Rufinamide has no structural similarities with other antiepileptic drugs. This makes it a promising alternative if needed. The European Medicines Agency (EMEA) approved rufinamide in 2007 as an "orphan drug" for the treatment of Lennox-Gastaut syndrome. It is approved in the United States, but not yet in Canada. Rufinamide is now widely available in several European countries and the United States. Note: see also the section "Orphan Drugs" in the front matter of this book.

HOW DOES RUFINAMIDE WORK?
WHAT IS THE CORRECT DOSAGE?

The basic antiepileptic effect mechanism of rufinamide is based on its influence on the sodium ion channels. This mechanism distinguishes itself from conventional antiepileptic drugs that also impact the sodium channels, such as carbamazepine, phenytoin, and lamotrigine. The difference is that the rapid electrical stream through the cell membrane is not suppressed, but instead its duration is extended. As such, it extends the refractory period further, which reduces the readiness for a new seizure. Rufinamide is available in dosage units of 100 mg, 200 mg, and 400 mg. In general it is administered twice daily, in the morning and evening. As the body absorbs the medication differently when taken with or without meals, it is important that you maintain a consistent pattern. Inconsistent administration will lead to spikes or valleys in your blood levels, impacting the seizure risk or the risk of side effects. Customarily, treatment is initiated with a single dosage of 200 mg, at times 400 mg.

The dosage can be increased in intervals of several days by 200 mg. This step-up rate can be modulated. The final dosage will be determined individually. The maximum dosage is 3,200 mg. In individual cases, and with good tolerance and effect, your doctor may recommend a higher dosage. As the concurrent administration of valproic acid slows the discharge of rufinamide and increases rufinamide levels in the blood, a slow introduction to rufinamide is necessary, especially in patients weighing less than 30 kg. Rufinamide blood levels can be reduced with the concurrent use of the enzyme-inducing medication phenytoin.

WHAT DO WE TREAT WITH
RUFINAMIDE, AND HOW
EFFECTIVE IS IT?

Rufinamide has been approved as an adjunct drug for patients 4 years of age and older who are being treated for Lennox-Gastaut syndrome. The adjustment phase should be managed by an epilepsy expert with a neurology and/or pediatric background. Lennox-Gastaut syndrome is typically manifested, with very few exceptions, between 3 and 5 years of age. This is seen as one of the most difficult-to-treat epilepsies. Seizures leading to falls, myoclonic seizures, absences, complex partial, focal, and tonic-clonic seizures are common. A controlled study with 138 adults and children from age 4 to 37 years and afflicted with Lennox-Gastaut syndrome showed these results: with rufinamide administered as an adjunct medication, in addition to one to three main anti-epileptic drugs, a significant reduction of seizures with falls (42%) was achieved with a daily dosage of 45m/kg/day when compared to the control group, which received a placebo. In addition, a 31.2% reduction of all other types of seizures was observed. The frequency of absences was reduced by 50.6%. The severity of seizures was reduced by 53.4%. A follow-up long-term study showed these observations as stable.

WHAT DO YOU NEED TO KNOW ABOUT THE SIDE EFFECTS OF RUFINAMIDE?

Information on how rufinamide is tolerated is based on the above-mentioned study and additional observations of more than 1,000 patients who were treated with rufinamide prior to official approval. One in ten patients treated with rufinamide discontinued the therapy due to side effects. The most frequent side effects that led to the discontinuation of the therapy were rashes and vomiting.

Brain and Psyche

One out of four patients treated with rufinamide reported sleepiness as a symptom (FP/S). This symptom was temporary and mild.

At times a slow-down of the adjustment phase or an adjustment of the dosage brought the desired relief. In long-term studies, sleepiness was rarely reported as a symptom. However, sleepiness, exhaustion, and headaches were reported more often. In contrast, the frequency of the above-mentioned side effects was comparable to the control group given a placebo. All side effects were rare, not severe, and temporary. In light of the fact that rufinamide is still a new medication, your personal observations are very valuable and should be reported to your consulting physician.

Allergies and Skin

Occasional skin rashes were observed during the adjustment phase. This side effect has often led to the discontinuation of treatment. Rashes should immediately be reported to your specialist.

Again, we want to bring to your attention that rufinamide is a new medication; as such, not all side effects are yet known. You should therefore discuss all unwanted physical and mental symptoms with your physician, including those that are not noted on the product description.

Blood

Not known.

Bone

Not known.

Gastrointestinal Tract and Internal Organs

Vomiting was the most reported side effect and occurred in 21.6% of the patients treated with rufinamide. If persistent, discuss this side effect with your specialist (FP/S).

Heart

Rufinamide may lead to a prolongation of the QT interval on the electrocardiogram (EKG). An EKG is therefore recommended before treatment, and caution is advised in concurrent medications with other QT-interval influencing drugs such as lamotrigine.

Interaction with Other Drugs

Rufinamide may interact with other antiepileptic drugs. We know that valproate markedly increases the serum concentration of rufinamide, and that rufinamide may increase the serum levels of other antiepileptic drugs such as phenytoin.

Contraception, Pregnancy, and Breast Feeding

Although rufinamide, unlike other antiepileptic drugs, does not accelerate metabolic activity and may even suppress it, it is known that it decreases the level of birth control hormones in the blood. This means that prevention from an unwanted pregnancy, managed by the contraceptive pill, is not certain while taking rufinamide at the same time. Your doctor or gynecologist may in that case recommend other forms of contraception. Epilepsy minimally increases the risk of birth defects even without antiepileptic drugs. The risk is not increased while being treated with this antiepileptic medication. Animal experiments have not provided indicators of fetal damage due to rufinamide. Should you become pregnant while already on rufinamide therapy, do not discontinue the medication on your own accord. This may lead to an increase in seizures, which could present a greater danger to your baby than rufinamide itself. Consult instead a specialist immediately, and discuss the further course of action.

We have now thoroughly informed you about the rare but possible side effects of rufinamide. You should be aware that your doctor selected this medication because it currently presents the best possible treatment for your epilepsy, with minimal side effects.

Successful rufinamide therapy is only possible if you take the medication as directed. Only in this way will you avoid large fluctuations of the drug in your blood. Once full dosage has been established and optimal blood levels have been reached, the rate of seizures should go down. If this is not the case, seek the advice of your epilepsy specialist immediately.

Stiripentol

Dear patient,

Your doctor has prescribed stiripentol for the treatment of your epilepsy. Based on years of observations in the management of epilepsies, we want to inform you about the effects and side effects of this medication. In addition to the standard product description that came with your medication, we share with you our expertise in a simple and understandable format. Stiripentol was first identified as an active agent in 1978 and was further developed in France in 1980. In December 2007, the European Medicines Agency (EMEA) approved stiripentol as an "orphan drug" for the treatment of Dravet syndrome (in Canada it is only available through a special access program). Stiripentol has been approved in selected countries as an orphan drug. Dravet syndrome is also known as severe myoclonic epilepsy of infancy (SMEI). It is used in combination therapy for the treatment of generalized tonic-clonic seizures associated with Dravet syndrome. This applies especially in cases where standard medications such as clobazam and valproate did not provide sufficient relief. The information here is not intended to replace the product description that came with your medication. Instead, you should read it thoroughly to filter out information that pertains to you. This guide provides solid advance information to initiate a detailed consultation with your doctor.

HOW DOES STIRIPENTOL WORK?
WHAT IS THE CORRECT DOSAGE?

Stiripentol affects the inhibitory neurotransmitter GABA (gamma-aminobutyric acid), offering seizure suppressing characteristics. While, on one hand, it increases the release of GABA, it also stretches the open interval of the sodium channels that occur at the binding site of GABA in the brain. In addition, stiripentol restrains some of the liver enzymes (cytochrome-P450-isoenzymes) that are active in the breakdown of other antiepileptic drugs. As such, it indirectly suppresses seizures. Stiripentol is available in capsule and water-soluble powder form, in dosage units of 250 mg and 500 mg. The dosage, in combination with clobazam and valproate, is based on an individual's weight. The suggested ratio is 50 mg per kg per day. The target dosage should be reached within three days. Stiripentol can be administered two to three times daily, with meals.

Stiripentol should not be taken in conjunction with milk products, carbonated drinks, caffeine, or drinks containing theophyllines. Based on stiripentol's impact on different cytochrome-P450-isoenzymes, a careful monitoring of accompanying medication in the serum plasma levels is recommended. In some cases it may become necessary to reduce the accompanying medication if related but unwanted side effects occur.

WHAT DO WE TREAT WITH
STIRIPENTOL, AND HOW
EFFECTIVE IS IT?

Stiripentol has been approved as an adjunct medication for the treatment of patients with Dravet syndrome. Dravet syndrome is a severe form of epilepsy that was first described in 1978 by Charlotte Dravet. This severe childhood epilepsy has its onset between 3 and 9 months of age. Seizures occur with fever and may be expressed in asymmetric tonic-clonic or generalized seizures.

During further progression of this illness, additional seizure types such as myoclonic and focal seizures as well as absences may occur. The main cause of Dravet syndrome is a mutant gene that is required by a protein within the neural membrane in the sodium channel. Key studies providing the basis for the approval of stiripentol were conducted in France and Italy. These studies compared the efficacy of stiripentol, when given with clobazam and valproate, against data collected from the control group who were given a placebo. A total of 65 patients, ranging in age from 3 to 18 years, who suffered a minimum of four tonic-clonic attacks per months, were studied. All patients were already being treated with clobazam and valproate.

The French study showed a significant reduction of attacks by 71.4% within the stiripentol group (experimental group), whereas the placebo (control) group showed a reduction of only 5%. The results of an Italian study were similar. The efficacy of stiripentol over a 3-month research period was also documented. Ninety percent of the test subjects in the French study were observed for another 25 months. The study showed that 57% of the patients observed had a reduction in attacks of 50%. So far, over 1,000 patients have been treated with stiripentol. Another study showed that stiripentol is also effective with focal epilepsy. The small sample size could demonstrate a statistically significant advantage against a placebo group.

WHAT DO YOU NEED TO KNOW ABOUT THE SIDE EFFECTS OF STIRIPENTOL?

Brain and Psyche

Observations attributed the following side effects to stiripentol therapy: sleepiness, numbness, irritability, excitability, restlessness, aggressiveness, unsteady gate, and muscle fatigue. Based on the somewhat limited experience with stiripentol, you should visit your doctor at once if any of the above symptoms concern you. It may become necessary to also consult a specialist (FP/S). As mentioned, such symptoms may also be due to other antiepileptic medications (given in combination therapy) medications.

Allergies and Skin

These are not known yet. However, it is ever so important that if any symptoms on skin or mucous membranes appear, you contact your family physician, and if more questions remain unanswered, that you consult the specialist (FP/S).

Blood

Some patients in the controlled studies showed noticeable changes in their blood count. Mainly a reduction of white blood cells or platelets was observed. Occasionally, an increase of the eosinophil white blood cells was described, which may also be increased during allergic reactions. In such cases, your (FP/S) family doctor will consult the epilepsy specialist and discuss a further course of action. Any significant change in your blood profile should be discussed with your specialist.

Bone

Not known.

Gastrointestinal Tract and Internal Organs

Frequently observed side effects are loss of appetite and weight loss. In the event of significant weight loss, a major adjustment, or a discontinuation, of the therapy may have to be considered. In some cases, weight gain has been observed.

In some cases, elevated gamma-GT values were observed (mainly in combination therapy with carbamazepine). Significant side effects have not been documented. In general, these elevated levels are harmless and do not require action. However, your epilepsy specialist should be consulted.

Heart

Not known.

Interaction with Other Drugs

Caution is advised with stiripentol if it is to be used in combination with medication that is metabolized with the liver enzymes CYP2C19 (i.e., citalopram, omeprazol) or CYP3A4 (i.e., HIV protease suppressor, some antihistamines, chlorpheniram, sodium channel blockers, oral contraceptives, and codeine). Reciprocal effects with theophylline may also occur. Medications that are metabolized by the isoenzyme CYP2D6 (i.e., some beta blockers, antidepressants, psychopharmaceutical drugs, and pain medications) may increase in the blood serum due to the enzyme-suppressing effect of stiripentol.

If not absolutely essential, stiripentol **should not** be combined with the following medications.

1. Ergoalkaloids: ergotamine, dihydroergotamine, due to the risk of ergotism, which reduces blood flow to hands and feet, possibly causing tissue damage.
2. Cisapride, halofantrine, pimozid, chinidine, and bepridil, due to an increased risk of cardiac arrhythmias.
3. Immunosuppressive drugs such as tacrolimus, cyclosporine, and sirolismus may also appear in increased levels in the blood stream.
4. Statins, due to dosage-dependent damage to muscle tissue (rhabdomyolysis).

Regarding the combination of stiripentol with other antiepileptic drugs, dosage determination of the associated additional medication and monitoring of the blood serum are needed. The enzyme-suppressing characteristics will lower the metabolic rate of medications such as phenobarbital, primidone, phenytoin, carbamazepine, clobazam, diazepam, and ethosuximide. The potential of reciprocal effects with valproic acid is small, suggesting that a dosage adjustment here is generally not required. The same applies to topiramate and levetiracetam. Again, we want to bring to your attention that stiripentol is a new medication; as such, not all side effects are yet known. You should therefore discuss all unwanted physical and mental symptoms with your physician, including those that are not noted on the product description.

Contraception, Pregnancy, and Breast Feeding

Since stiripentol does not accelerate liver metabolic activity, and may even suppress it, contraceptive protection with oral contraceptives is not affected, though further research is needed to clarify this issue. Epilepsy minimally increases the risk of birth defects even without this antiepileptic drug. The risk is not increased while being treated with antiepileptic medication. Animal experiments have not provided indicators of fetal damage due to stiripentol. Should you become pregnant while on stiripentol, you should not discontinue the medication on your own accord, as this could lead to an increase in seizures, presenting a greater harm to your baby than stiripentol itself. Consult a specialist immediately, and discuss the further course of action.

We have now thoroughly informed you about the rare but possible side effects of stiripentol. You should be aware that your doctor selected this medication because it currently presents the best possible treatment for your epilepsy, with minimal side effects.

Successful stiripentol therapy is only possible if you take the medication as directed. Only in this way will you avoid large fluctuations of the drug in your blood. Once full dosage has been established and optimal blood levels have been reached, the rate of seizures should go down. If this is not the case, seek the advice of your epilepsy specialist immediately.

Tiagabine

How Does
It Work?
What Are
the Side
Effects?

Dear patient,

Your doctor has prescribed tiagabine for the treatment of your epilepsy. Based on years of observations in the management of epilepsies, we want to inform you about the effects and side effects of this medication. In addition to the standard product description that came with your medication, we share with you our expertise in a simple and understandable format. Tiagabine was approved in Europe in 1996, and short after in the United States in 1997 as adjunct medication for patients with refractory focal epilepsies. It is not approved in Canada, but is available through a special access program. Years of clinical observations and trials have given us a good scope on its effectiveness and its side effects. The information here is not intended to replace the product description that came with your medication. Instead, you should read it thoroughly to filter out information that pertains to you. The following text offers you thorough advance information to provide a good base for a detailed discussion with your doctor.

HOW DOES TIAGABINE WORK?
WHAT IS THE CORRECT DOSAGE?

The composition of tiagabine does not compare with other antiepileptic drugs. The medication engages the metabolism of the seizure-suppressing neurotransmitter GABA (gamma-aminobutyric acid). Tiagabine prevents the re-entry of GABA from the intercellular space back into the cell. This results in a prolonged seizure-suppressing potential. Most studies are based on daily dosages of 30 mg to 80 mg. The initially required and tolerable dosage should be determined together with your epilepsy specialist (FP/S). Tiagabine must be gradually stepped up to the target dose. This will reduce the risk of side effects. Because of the short half-life time, it is recommended that it be taken three times daily. The medication is available in tablet form in dosage units of 5 mg, 10 mg, and 15 mg.

WHAT DO WE TREAT WITH TIAGABINE, AND HOW EFFECTIVE IS IT?

So far, tiagabine has been used on patients to treat focal seizures and large (grand mal) seizures, where traditional medications did not provide the required relief in seizure frequency and severity. Of patients who received tiagabine in addition to preceding medication, approximately 25% to 40% of these patients experienced a reduction in seizure frequency by at least 50%. The effective dosage for adults was 30 mg to 80 mg of tiagabine daily. The medication was given in combination with carbamazepine or phenytoin. The approval of tiagabine is so far limited to be used as adjunct medication for patients with difficult-to-treat focal epilepsies.

WHAT DO YOU NEED TO KNOW ABOUT THE SIDE EFFECTS OF TIAGABINE?

Side effects forcing a discontinuation of this therapy are rare, but as the medication is still new, not enough conclusive data are available. Therefore you should address any unwanted physical or mental side effects that you notice with your physician, even if these are not mentioned in the product description. Any further course of action should only be determined with your doctor. Unskilled management, such as by discontinuing the medication, could lead to a dangerous increase in seizure frequency.

Brain and Psyche

Especially after treatment initiation and during the adjustment phase, during which time the daily dosage is still gradually stepped up, fatigue, dizziness, and an unsteady gate may occur (FP/S). Less frequent reports were of eye tremors (nystagmus), nervousness, shaking, depression, mood swings, confusion and headaches. Should the above-mentioned symptoms continue, consult your doctor, and in case of greater severity your specialist (FP/S). Quick relief is often obtained with a dosage reduction or a redistribution of the daily dosage. When symptoms of dizziness or double vision occur, you may ask a friend or relative if you have nystagmus, or "shaking eye." Your doctor will gladly explain how you can diagnose this. Frequently, patients who are being treated with antiepileptic medication report impeded physical performance and concentration ability. Research has so far not determined with certainty to what degree this medication is, or may be, responsible for this. Observations to this date suggest that tiagabine has no measurable negative impact on intelligence, memory, or attention abilities. However, it cannot be assumed with certainty that in individual cases undesirable symptoms will not appear. If you suspect any physical or intellectual impairment, consult a specialist. Perhaps relief can be achieved with a minor adjustment in the treatment management.

Allergies and Skin

Only very rarely, and in isolated cases, were skin rashes attributed to tiagabine. However, it is ever so important that, if any symptoms on skin or mucous membranes appear, you contact your family physician, and if more questions remain unanswered, that you consult the specialist (FP/S).

Blood

Not known.

Bone

Not known.

Gastrointestinal Tract and Internal Organs

Nausea, vomiting, and diarrhea have been reported more frequently during tiagabine therapy when compared to a placebo control group. In such cases, see your family doctor, who may send you to a specialist (FP/S). Persistent sore throat, stomach pain, and black stools have been occasionally reported. So far, there are no indicators pointing to serious side effects on the liver, cardiovascular system, or the blood-building systems (bone marrow). Again, we want to bring to your attention that tiagabine is a new medication; as such, not all side effects are yet known. You should therefore discuss all unwanted physical and mental symptoms with your physician, including those that are not noted on the product description.

Heart

Not known.

Interaction with Other Drugs

Tiagabine does not influence the serum concentrations of other drugs in a clinically relevant way. Vice versa, enzyme-inducing antiepileptic drugs such as carbamazepine, phenytoin, phenobarbital, or oxcarbazepine may decrease the serum concentration of tiagabine. It may be necessary for the specialist (S) to increase the dosage under such circumstances in order to improve antiepileptic efficacy.

Contraception, Pregnancy, and Breast Feeding

Tiagabine, unlike the older antiepileptic medications, does not accelerate the metabolic rate of the liver. In agreement with a reciprocal effect study, it was shown that the hormonal content and contraceptive protection of the birth control pill were not affected during concurrent administration of tiagabine. Epilepsy minimally increases the risk of birth defects even without antiepileptic drugs. Animal experiments have not provided indicators of fetal damage due to tiagabine. Since the drug has so far only been used in combination therapy, insufficient human data is available. Thus we do not recommend taking tiagabine during pregnancy and breast feeding.

We have now thoroughly informed you about the rare but possible side effects of tiagabine. You should be aware that your doctor selected this medication because it currently presents the best possible treatment for your epilepsy, with minimal side effects.

Successful tiagabine therapy is only possible if you take the medication as directed. Only in this way will you avoid large fluctuations of the drug in your blood. Once full dosage has been established and optimal blood levels have been reached, the rate of seizures should go down. If this is not the case, seek the advice of your epilepsy specialist immediately.

Topiramate | How Does It Work? What Are the Side Effects?

Dear patient,

Your doctor has prescribed topiramate for the treatment of your epilepsy.

Based on years of observations in the management of epilepsies, we want to inform you about the effects and side effects of this medication. In addition to the standard product description that came with your medication, we share with you our expertise in a simple and understandable format. The information here is not intended to replace the product description that came with your medication. Instead, you should read it thoroughly to filter out information that pertains to you. This guide provides solid advance information to initiate a detailed consultation with your doctor. Topiramate was approved in many European countries, in the United States (1996) and in Canada (1997) as add-on therapy in refractory focal epilepsy, followed by monotherapy approval in 2005. Extensive knowledge about this medication was collected internationally in clinical trials. Years of clinical observations provided a good scope on its effectiveness and its side effects.

HOW DOES TOPIRAMATE WORK?
WHAT IS THE CORRECT DOSAGE?

The composition of topiramate is unlike common antiepileptic drugs. Its efficacy is believed to be based on multiple mechanisms. Topiramate stabilizes the electrical activity of the neural membranes and as such reduces the electrical excitation potential. In addition, this medication engages the metabolism of the seizure-suppressing neurotransmitter GABA (gamma-aminobutyric acid). The resulting higher concentration in the intercellular space is assumed to have a seizure-suppressing effect. Initial studies were conducted with daily dosages ranging from 200 mg to 600 mg. However, the observations were recorded during add-on treatments in difficult-to-treat cases.

More recent studies showed the efficacy of topiramate in mono-therapy with a small daily dosage of only 50 mg. The target topiramate dosage should be determined by an epilepsy specialist (S). Due to metabolic characteristics of topiramate, we recommend that the daily dosage be administered in two to three intervals. The medication is available in tablet form, in dosage units of 25 mg, 100 mg, and 200 mg, and in sprinkle capsules of 15 mg and 25 mg.

WHAT DO WE TREAT WITH
TOPIRAMATE, AND HOW
EFFECTIVE IS IT?

Topiramate was initially used to treat patients with partial and secondarily generalized epileptic seizures who did not respond to other epileptic medications. Patients received topiramate, in addition to already established medication. About 50% of these patients experienced a reduction in the frequency rate of seizures by half. The effective dosage in those days, for adults, was 200 mg to 600 mg daily. Indications are that topiramate can also be effective with non-focal epilepsies. Lower daily dosages of 100 mg to 200 mg have also been effective with newly diagnosed epilepsies.

Older patients appear to be a well-suited target group. Often dosages between 50 mg and 100 mg are sufficient. Side effects were also significantly less than was shown in earlier studies with higher dosages and in adjunct therapy. Topiramate also has been approved as a prophylactic medication to prevent migraine attacks.

WHAT DO YOU NEED TO KNOW ABOUT THE SIDE EFFECTS OF TOPIRAMATE?

Since this product has only been available for a few years, no long-term observations are at hand. Thus, you should report any undesired physical or mental symptoms that you notice while taking topiramate to your doctor, even if these are not mentioned in the product description (FP/S). This applies to any related complaints. Unskilled handling or discontinuing the medication on your own accord increases the risk of further seizures.

Brain and Psyche

Especially after treatment initiation and during the adjustment phase, during which time the daily dosage is still gradually being stepped up, fatigue, dizziness, an unsteady gait, headache, mood swings, eye tremors (nystagmus), and slurred speech may occur. Should such symptoms continue, consult your doctor, and maybe even your specialist (FP/S). Quick relief is often obtained with a dosage reduction or a redistribution of the daily dose. Should these symptoms continue, discontinuation of the medication may be needed. When symptoms of dizziness or double vision occur, you may ask a friend or relative if you have nystagmus ("shaking eye"). Your doctor will gladly explain how you can diagnose this. Less frequent side effects may be increased nervousness, mood swings, confusion, psychosis and hallucinations, panic fears, speech and syntax impairment. Gradual dosage increase during the adjustment phase reduces the risk of side effects. Getting to the recommended daily target dosage of 200 mg takes several weeks. In cases when a quick result is needed, due to frequent seizures, topiramate can be introduced at a faster pace. Be patient and don't become discouraged. Frequently, patients who are being treated with antiepileptic medication report impeded physical performance and concentration ability. Research has so far not determined with certainty to what degree this medication may be responsible for this. Observations suggest that topiramate may have a negative impact on memory, speech fluency, response times, and attention abilities in some patients. However, no undesirable symptoms occur in many patients taking this drug. When in doubt, consult a specialist. Relief can often be achieved with a minor adjustment to the treatment program.

Allergies and Skin

Skin rashes have reported in conjunction with topiramate therapy. Allergic reactions to topiramate have so far not been observed. However, it is important that if any skin or mucous membrane symptom occurs, you should contact your family physician, and if more questions remain unanswered, that you consult the specialist (FP/S).

Blood

Not known.

Bone

Not known.

Gastrointestinal Tract and Internal Organs

Kidney stones developed in 1.5% of patients treated with topiramate. This occurs especially if there is a tendency to develop kidney stones in your family. Regular blood and urine screens allow for an early diagnosis and subsequent treatment. Dosage-related weight loss has been observed in 10–15% of patients. Nothing points to serious side effects in the cardiovascular system. In isolated cases, increased intraocular pressure has been recorded. Reduced ability to perspire (sweat) and a slight overheating of the body were reported. Consult your doctor immediately should eye pressure, headaches, or a limited and a reduced amount of heat tolerance be noted, especially during athletic activities (FP/S).

Heart

Not known.

Interaction with Other Drugs

Topiramate may increase the serum concentration of phenytoin. Enzyme-inducing antiepileptic drugs such as carbamazepine, phenytoin, or phenobarbital may decrease the serum concentration of topiramate. It may be necessary for the specialist (S) to increase the dosage under such circumstances to improve the antiepileptic efficacy.

Contraception, Pregnancy, and Breast Feeding

Contraceptive protection may be diminished, as topiramate reduces the efficacy of the contraceptive pill. Epilepsy minimally increases the risk of birth defects even without antiepileptic drugs. Animal research has not pointed to any subsequent birth defect. Should you become pregnant while on topiramate, you should not discontinue the medication on your own accord, as this could lead to an increase in attacks, which could present a greater harm to your baby than topiramate itself. Consult instead a specialist immediately, and discuss the further course of action.

We have now thoroughly informed you about the rare but possible side effects of topiramate. You should be aware that your doctor selected this medication because it currently presents the best possible treatment for your epilepsy, with minimal side effects.

Successful topiramate therapy is only possible if you take the medication as directed. Only in this way will you avoid large fluctuations of the drug in your blood. Once full dosage has been established and optimal blood levels have been reached, the rate of seizures should go down. If this is not the case, seek the advice of your epilepsy specialist immediately.

Valproic Acid/ Valproate/Divalproex Sodium

How Does It Work? What Are the Side Effects?

Dear patient,

Your doctor has prescribed valproic acid (or valproate or divalproex sodium) for the treatment of your epilepsy. Based on years of observations in the management of epilepsies, we want to inform you about the effects and side effects of this medication. In addition to the standard product description that came with your medication, we share with you our expertise in a simple and understandable format. This information is not intended to replace the product description that came with your medication. Instead, you should read it thoroughly to filter out information that pertains to you. The following text offers you thorough advance information to provide a good base for a detailed discussion with your doctor.

HOW DOES VALPROIC ACID WORK? WHAT IS THE CORRECT DOSAGE?

Chemists have understood valproic acid for more than 100 years. However, its efficacy in the treatment for epileptic seizures was noticed by accident in the 1960s. The way in which this antiepileptic medication works is not yet understood. Multiple mechanisms are likely. It is very likely that it increases the inhibitory neurotransmitter GABA (gamma-aminobutyric acid). In addition, valproate acid also stabilizes the neural membranes, lowering the excitation threshold. This prevents a simultaneous electrical discharge of a cluster of cells and thus reduces the potential of a seizure to occur.

The common dosage is based on 20 mg to 30 mg per kg of body weight. Depending on tolerability and efficacy, individual cases may warrant a significantly higher dosage. Please be patient! The desired results are sometimes not noticed until several weeks have passed. The metabolic characteristics allow a one-time daily administration. Occasionally, multiple dosages within a day are necessary. The above-mentioned products contain valproic acid, or its sodium salts (divalproex sodium), in several dosage units. Tablets of divalproex sodium are available in 125 mg, 250 mg, 450 mg, and 500 mg. Valproic acid is also available as capsules of 250 mg and 500 mg, as well as lozenge and liquid solution (syrup: 250 mg/5 ml). It is now also available in intravenous form, used in case of status epilepticus.

WHAT DO WE TREAT WITH VALPROIC ACID, AND HOW EFFECTIVE IS IT?

Initially, valproic acid was used to treat patients with absences, myoclonic seizures (generalized muscle jerks), and grand mal seizures (all of them considered generalized seizure types), and has long been a medication of first choice for these forms of epilepsy. The medication has long been used to treat a broad band of epilepsies. As such, it is also used successfully for the treatment of focal epilepsy and has also become the primary medication for this condition. Valproic acid is also available for injection and can thus be administered in cases where oral administration is not suitable. Its active ingredient is also effective in the prophylactic treatment of migraine attacks, as well as for the therapy of manic depressive disorders.

WHAT DO YOU NEED TO KNOW ABOUT THE SIDE EFFECTS OF VALPROIC ACID?

Brain and Psyche

During therapy with valproic acid, dizziness, unsteady gate, slurred speech, and double vision may occur. However, these side effects occur much less often than with other antiepileptic medications (FP/S). When symptoms of dizziness or double vision occur, you may ask a friend or relative to check for "eye tremor" (nystagmus). Your doctor will gladly explain how you can diagnose this. With larger dosages, shaking of the hands (tremor) can appear, even when resting, and is aggravated by targeted motor activity. Rarely will you experience exhaustion and lack of motivation, or delirious perception. Should such complaints reach a level of concern, consult your doctor or specialist. Normally, these bothersome but harmless symptoms disappear after the adjustment phase or after a minor dosage correction. Extremely rare during valproic acid therapy are fatigue, lethargy, or impaired consciousness, occurring a few days after treatment has begun. This is known as valproic acid encephalopathy. This syndrome disappears after discontinuing the medication within hours or days. In cases of extreme fatigue, you should immediately consult your epilepsy specialist (S/ED).

Frequently, patients who are being treated with antiepileptic medication report impeded physical performance and concentration ability. Research has so far not determined with certainty to what degree this medication may be responsible for this. Observations to this date suggest that valproic acid may have a negative impact on intelligence, memory, and attention abilities, but only in a small proportion of patients. Relief can often be achieved with a minor adjustment in drug dosage.

Allergies and Skin

Allergic reactions and skin problems are unusual with valproic acid. However, if any skin or mucous membrane symptoms occur, it is important that you contact your family physician, and if more questions remain unanswered, that you consult the specialist (FP/S).

Blood

Valproic acid affects the coagulation of your blood. Most of the time this is of little clinical significance. Skin bleeding, nosebleeds, or larger bruises may be indicators of coagulation issues. Consult your doctor immediately to have this addressed. Combining valproic acid with aspirin or other acetylsalicylic acids is not recommended due to its impact on blood coagulation, and surgeons should, prior to commencing surgery, be informed about the presence of valproic acid, so that coagulation tests can be performed beforehand, and any bleeding tendencies are understood and proactively managed. Occasionally, decreases of white or red blood cells or of thrombocytes (cells that promote normal blood clotting) may happen; this needs to be carefully watched and controlled by the specialist (S), who will decide whether it is possible to continue the therapy.

Bone

Although the mechanism is not completely understood, there are some hints that with valproic acid, bone density may be reduced over years. This is a possibility with many antiepileptic drugs, so the specialist will be fully aware of the need to watch the possibility of that side effect carefully (S).

Gastrointestinal Tract and Internal Organs

Patients treated with valproic acid rarely report stomach pain, malaise (a general ill feeling), or nausea. Thanks to the wide range of valproic acid–based medications, it should be possible to find one that suits you. In the early days of using valproic acid, about 20 years ago, serious problems occurred in rare cases in the treatment of severely mentally handicapped children, who were concurrently being treated with other medications, and some deaths were reported due to acute liver failure and, in even rarer cases, pancreatitis. This observation led to the recommendation that during the adjustment phase, especially with children, frequent laboratory tests are requested. Initially, these are run every 2 weeks and then are followed up at longer intervals. The following complaints should be addressed immediately by a specialist (FP/S): loss of appetite, consciousness issues, an acquired rejection of previously liked meals, nausea, apathy, vomiting, edema, prolonged bleeding, and an increase in seizure frequency. Such complaints have sometimes occurred in conjunction with febrile infections, but laboratory tests at the onset of the therapy have helped drastically to reduce these incidences. Increased appetite and weight gain have also been reported during therapy. Should the appetite not be successfully controlled, dosage reduction may be required. The weight gain is reversible after the adjustment phase. The same applies to occasionally observed hair loss, which ceased with a subsequent dosage correction. In general, you should see your family doctor first if any side effects are noticed. If the cause for your complaints cannot be isolated, you may be asked to see a specialist.

Heart

Not known.

Interaction with Other Drugs

Valproic acid has numerous interactions with other drugs. In principle, it elevates the serum concentration of other drugs. The serum concentration of phenobarbital may rise. The concentration of carbamazepine epoxide, a metabolite that is sometimes responsible for tolerability problems under carbamazepine, increases. Since valproic acid may diminish the protein-binding rate of carbamazepine and phenytoin, the free fractions of those antiepileptic drugs may rise and cause side effects. Lamotrigine levels may show a fourfold increase. Enzyme-inducing drugs like carbamazepine, phenytoin, phenobarbital, oxcarbazepine, and also felbamate may decrease the serum concentration of valproic acid. It may be necessary for the specialist (S) to interfere therapeutically if such interactions impair the efficacy and tolerability of the treatment with valproic acid.

Contraception, Pregnancy, and Breast Feeding

Frequent birth defects have been reported during valproic acid therapy, including especially cases of neural development disorder (open spine, spina bifida) (FP/S). The risk of such birth defects is estimated at 1–2% in mothers with epilepsy and on valproate, and is much higher (by a factor of 10 to 20) than pregnancies in healthy mothers. Other birth defects affecting skeletal structures, the heart, and the urogenital tract also occurred more frequently during valproic acid therapy. The risk is reduced if valproic acid is taken as monotherapy, given in the lowest possible dosage, and given over several administrations during the day. Address pregnancy, or the desire to become pregnant, with your doctor as early as possible to allow for better therapy management. It is recommended that prior to conception and in the early stages of pregnancy, folic acid be administered (ask your specialist about this). Under no circumstances should you discontinue the medication on your own. This may have unpredictable consequences for you and your child. As only 3% of valproic acid is carried into breast milk, breast feeding is not a concern. Consult your epilepsy specialist for more information. Valproic acid does not accelerate the metabolic activity in the liver, and as such does not impede contraceptive protection.

We have now thoroughly informed you about the rare but possible side effects of valproic acid. You should be aware that your doctor selected this medication because it currently presents the best possible treatment for your epilepsy, with minimal side effects.

Successful valproic acid therapy is only possible if you take the medication as directed. Only in this way will you avoid large fluctuations of the drug in your blood. Once full dosage has been established and optimum blood levels have been reached, the rate of seizures should go down. If this is not the case, seek the advice of your epilepsy specialist immediately.

Vigabatrin | How Does It Work? What Are the Side Effects?

Dear patient,

Your doctor has prescribed vigabatrin for the treatment of your epilepsy. Based on years of observations in the management of epilepsies, we want to inform you about the effects and side effects of this medication. In addition to the standard product description that came with your medication, we share with you our expertise in a simple and understandable format. Vigabatrin has been clinically tested for a long time and was first approved in Canada in 1994. The information here is not intended to replace the product description that came with your medication. Instead, you should read it thoroughly to filter out information that pertains to you. The following text provides solid advance information to initiate a detailed consultation with your doctor.

HOW DOES VIGABATRIN WORK? WHAT IS THE CORRECT DOSAGE?

Chemically, vigabatrin is closely related to GABA (gamma-aminobutyric acid). GABA is a neurotransmitter in the central nervous system (CNS), which suppresses the excitability of neurons. Vigabatrin increases the GABA concentrations in the brain, which reduces excitation of the neurons and subsequently reduces the occurrence of seizures. Most research is based on observations made with daily dosages of 1 to 3 grams. Clinical experience showed that larger dosages were also tolerated. The decision to further increase the dosage must be made as part of the therapy management by an epilepsy specialist (FP/S). In contrast to other medications, vigabatrin can be increased within a few days to the target dosage. The medication is available as a 500 mg coated tablet. The daily dosage should be administered twice daily. In individual cases, a three-time daily administration may be desired. In case of reduction of renal function, a lower dosage must be chosen and discussed with your treating physician. A concurrent administration of vigabatrin with phenytoin may lead to lower levels of active phenytoin in the blood (within a few weeks). A subsequent increase of phenytoin may become necessary when breakthrough seizures occur.

WHAT DO WE TREAT WITH VIGABATRIN, AND HOW EFFECTIVE IS IT?

Vigabatrin has been used in the past to treat patients with focal and secondarily generalized epileptic seizures. It was primarily tested for complex partial seizures (psychomotor seizures) and in those patients who did not respond to other antiepileptic medications. These patients were given vigabatrin, in addition to an already established drug treatment regime. With half of the patients a 50% reduction of seizure frequency was achieved. Seven percent became completely seizure free. In addition, efficacy in the treatment of Lennox-Gastaut syndrome and West syndrome has been documented. The dosage for children is 40–100 mg per kilo/body weight per day. Current approval is limited to adjunct administration for adult patients with difficult-to-treat partial epilepsy, and for children with partial seizures, as well as West syndrome and Lennox-Gastaut syndrome.

WHAT DO YOU NEED TO KNOW ABOUT THE SIDE EFFECTS OF VIGABATRIN?

Side effects forcing a discontinuation of the medication are rare— with the exception of specific changes to the visual field described below, which require dedicated and careful attention. Since this product has been available for only a few years, not as many observations are at hand as for drugs that have been used for decades. Thus you should report any undesired physical or mental symptoms that you notice while taking vigabatrin with your doctor, even if these are not mentioned in the product description (FP/S). This applies to any related complaints. Unskilled handling or discontinuing the medication on your own accord adds the risk of an increase in seizures.

Brain and Psyche

Fatigue symptoms may occur during vigabatrin therapy. On rare occasions, patients complain about dizziness and headaches. Unsteady gait, double vision, and eye tremors (nystagmus) have occurred in few cases. In the event of dizziness, ask a relative or friend to check if your eyes are "shaking." Your doctor calls this "nystagmus" and will gladly explain how to diagnose it. Nystagmus may indicate a slight over-dosage. Should the side effects continue, consult your family doctor (FP) at once, and if the severity is of concern to you, go directly to the specialist. Normally, these bothersome but harmless side effects are gone shortly after the adjustment period or after a minor dosage adjustment. Distinct interference with vision is a serious side effect. It has been known for only a few years that nearly one-third of patients treated with vigabatrin experience irreversible side effects to the visual fields (tunnel vision). It is suggested that this significant side effect is a characteristic of vigabatrin; it is extremely rare with other antiepileptic drugs.

This issue of vigabatrin-associated visual field defects is currently being intensively researched. It is recommended that prior to commencing therapy with vigabatrin an examination to check your visual field needs to be completed. This examination should subsequently be repeated every 3 months during the course of the therapy.

Some patients report exhaustion and depression. Rarely, psychoses and hallucinations have been observed. These symptoms are usually controllable with a small dosage correction. Patients who have a previous history of psychiatric disorders are considered to be particularly at risk for these symptoms. Should you have a history of these or related symptoms, inform your doctor. If these symptoms do occur, you should consult an epilepsy specialist without hesitation. This applies especially to children.

Vigabatrin may cause restlessness, nervousness, sleeplessness, and hyperactivity (FP/S). If these symptoms continue, immediately consult your caregiver. The bothersome but mostly harmless symptoms usually disappear shortly after the adjustment phase, or after a minor dosage correction. Frequently, patients who are being treated with antiepileptic medication report impeded physical performance and concentration ability. Research has so far not determined with certainty to what degree this medication is, or may be, responsible for this. Observations to this date suggest that vigabatrin has no measurable negative impact on intelligence, memory, or attention abilities. However, it cannot be assumed with certainty that in individual cases undesirable symptoms will not appear. If you suspect any physical or intellectual impairment, consult a specialist. Perhaps relief can be achieved with a minor adjustment in your treatment management.

Allergies and Skin

Allergies have so far not been reported. However, if any symptoms appear on skin or mucous membranes, it is very important that you contact your family physician, and if more questions remain unanswered, that you consult the specialist (FP/S).

Blood

In isolated cases, a reduction of the hemoglobin concentration (and in even rarer cases, the white blood cells) was observed. Therefore your doctor should initially check your blood count, especially if you have anemia. Discuss any changes with a specialist.

Bone

Not known.

Gastrointestinal Tract and Internal Organs

Occasionally, weight gain has been reported during vigabatrin therapy. Nausea, vomiting, stomach pain, loss of appetite, and constipation are rare. In such cases, consult your family doctor first. Your doctor will decide if you need to be referred to a specialist.

Occasionally, a drop-off of liver values (AST and ALT) was observed, but this is of no significance. Again, we want to bring to your attention that vigabatrin is a new medication; as such, not all side effects are yet known. You should therefore discuss all unwanted physical and mental symptoms with your physician, including those that are not noted on the product description.

Heart

So far, clinically relevant effects of vigabatrin have not been observed.

Interaction with Other Drugs

Vigabatrin may decrease the serum concentration of phenobarbital and especially of phenytoin.

Contraception, Pregnancy, and Breast Feeding

Vigabatrin, unlike older antiepileptic medications, does not accelerate the metabolic rate of the liver. In agreement with a reciprocal effect study, it was shown that the hormonal content and contraceptive protection of the birth control pill were not affected during concurrent administration of vigabatrin. Epilepsy minimally increases the risk of birth defects, even without antiepileptic drugs. The risk is not increased while being treated with antiepileptic medication. Animal experiments have not provided indicators of fetal damage due to vigabatrin. However, should you discover that you have become pregnant while on vigabatrin, you should not discontinue the medication on your own accord, as this could lead to an increase in seizures, which could present a greater danger to your baby than vigabatrin itself. Consult a specialist immediately, and discuss the further course of action.

We have now thoroughly informed you about the rare but possible side effects of vigabatrin. You should be aware that your doctor selected this medication because it currently presents the best possible treatment for your epilepsy, with minimal side effects.

Successful vigabatrin therapy is only possible if you take the medication as directed. Only in this way will you avoid large fluctuations of the drug in your blood. Once full dosage has been established and optimal blood levels have been reached, the rate of seizures should go down. If this is not the case, seek the advice of your epilepsy specialist immediately.

Zonisamide

How Does
It Work?
What Are
the Side
Effects?

Dear patient,

Your doctor has prescribed zonisamide for the treatment of your epilepsy. Based on years of observations in the management of epilepsies, we want to inform you about the effects and side effects of this medication. In addition to the standard product description that came with your medication, we share with you our expertise in a simple and understandable format.

Initially, zonisamide was approved in Japan in 1989, followed by the United States in 2000. Many other countries followed (e.g., Germany in 2005). It was initially approved for partial and secondarily generalized tonic-clonic seizures in adult patients, 18 years and older. Zonisamide is not yet approved in Canada but is available through a special access program. Long-term observations in Japan led to the extension of the original approval. It now also encompasses generalized epilepsies for children from the age of 1 year, as well as monotherapy treatment. Significant clinical studies, some covering duration of more than 10 years, are available.

A comprehensive assessment of its effectiveness and its side effects cannot be made for several years, as this medication is still considered comparatively new on the market. The information here is not intended to replace the product description that came with your medication. Instead, you should read it thoroughly to filter out information that pertains to you. The following text provides solid advance information to initiate a detailed consultation with your doctor.

HOW DOES ZONISAMIDE WORK? WHAT IS THE CORRECT DOSAGE?

Zonisamide possesses several antiepileptic mechanisms of actions. Like the antiepileptic drugs carbamazepine and phenytoin, it suppresses the voltage-dependent sodium channels of the neurons. By blocking the calcium channels and the potassium-dependent release of the excitatory amino acid glutamate, an over-reaction (excitation) is suppressed. In addition, zonisamide acts on the enzyme carbonic anhydrase. This mechanism is similar to the mechanism of topiramate. Zonisamide is a benzisooxazol derivative, like other antibiotic medications. Zonisamide is quickly absorbed by the body. Protein binding is known to be 40%, which means that only 60% of the administered medication is effective. Zonisamide is significantly not engaged in liver metabolism, and is excreted by the kidneys. Thus, there is no impact on internal hormones or other antiepileptic drugs metabolized in the liver. These, however, can impact the zonisamide concentrations in the blood. For example, in a combination with primidone, phenobarbital, phenytoin, and to a lesser degree valproic acid, the discharging of zonisamide is accelerated and as such the blood concentration lowered. In such cases, it is reasonable to increase the dosage of zonisamide in order to increase its treatment effect. On the other hand, a reduction of the above-mentioned medications, without changing the dosage of zonisamide, may achieve the desired result. This may increase some side effects but will improve its antiepileptic effect. Your doctor should weigh all options and assure that the optimal dosage for you is determined. Due to the long half-life of 63 hours, zonisamide can be taken twice daily, in the morning and in the evening. As a result, it may also take a few days for the drug level in the serum to stabilize at a "steady state." After the steady state is reached, you can determine how well the medication is tolerated. Comprehensive studies with dosages ranging from 300 mg to 600 mg are available. These dosages were both effective and well tolerated. There are also indicators that lower dosages of 200 mg showed desirable results. This in turn is likely to improve the tolerance of the medication even more. A recommendation as to which daily dosage will be effective cannot yet be made until further research has been completed. The individually required and tolerable dosage on zonisamide should finally be determined by your epilepsy specialist (FP/S).

Zonisamide should always be stepped up to the anticipated dosage gradually. A dosage of 2 × 25 mg during the first week of treatment is recommended. During the second week, the dosage can be increased to 2 × 100 mg. In the third week, 2 × 150 mg can be administered. Another variant is to administer 100 mg in the morning and 200 mg in the evening. A twice-daily schedule to reach the daily dosage is necessary and sufficient. The medication is currently available in tablet form. The dosage units are 20 mg, 50 mg, and 100 mg. The medication is currently approved for the treatment of focal epilepsy, with or without potential to a grand mal seizure. Reciprocal effects with other medications, such as anticoagulants or oral contraceptives, have not been shown and are not expected.

WHAT DO WE TREAT WITH ZONISAMIDE, AND HOW EFFECTIVE IS IT?

Zonisamide is approved for the treatment of adult patients with "partial" (focal) and secondarily generalized tonic-clonic seizures, where traditional treatments have failed to bring about the desired results. Several large and comprehensive studies conducted with patients suffering from difficult-to-treat epilepsy showed that add-on zonisamide therapy reduced the frequency of seizures by more than half in 30% of cases observed. These observations pointed to the strong efficacy of zonisamide. Good data suggest that zonisamide can be effective for a broad range of epilepsies, including generalized seizures. An approval extension for its use in a broader range of epilepsy has already been granted in Japan.

WHAT DO YOU NEED TO KNOW ABOUT THE SIDE EFFECTS OF ZONISAMIDE?

Due to the somewhat limited knowledge of side effects with zonisamide, every symptom you experience will be assumed to be a possible side effect. Should the effect continue, or increase in severity to be of concern, call your family doctor or epilepsy specialist. Side effects forcing a discontinuation of the medication are rare but require careful attention.

Brain and Psyche

During the adjustment phase of the therapy, especially if done quickly, symptoms such as fatigue, dizziness, lack of spontaneity, irritability, sleeplessness, depression, and concentration and memory challenges may occur. In the rarest cases, hallucination, unsteady gate, eye tremors (nystagmus), and slurry speech have been reported. Other typical side effects are pain sensitivities, such as pins-and-needles sensations (paresthesias), which will ease after a few weeks, and often fade altogether. These symptoms are bothersome but not dangerous. Normally, these mostly harmless symptoms disappear a short while after the adjustment phase, or after a minor dosage correction. Should some of these symptoms prevail even after a dosage adjustment, or if some of these symptoms are severe, a discontinuation of the medication might be considered. A gradually paced adjustment phase reduces the risk of the above-mentioned side effects. You need to be patient. Don't let this discourage you.

Allergies and Skin

On rare occasions, skin rashes and allergic reactions were reported in conjunction with zonisamide. Patients with a known sensitivity to sulfonamides should be cautious taking zonisamide. However, allergic skin reactions are rare. If any symptoms appear on skin or mucous membranes, it is important that you contact your family physician, and if more questions remain unanswered, that you consult the specialist (FP/S).

Blood

In rare, isolated cases (less than 1%), a reduction in hemoglobin and white cells and red blood cells was reported.

Bone

Not known.

Gastrointestinal Tract and Internal Organs

A significant portion of patients may experience weight loss. Interference with other organs has also been reported, but did not differ significantly from the observation of an untreated control group, who received a placebo.

Currently available studies report an increased risk of developing kidney stones. It is important to be proactive, and to assure that sufficient volume of liquids are given. If a family history of kidney stones is known, you must inform your doctor (FP/S). In that case, a switch of medication may be considered.

Heart

So far, there are no indicators of serious side effects.

Interaction with Other Drugs

Zonisamide hardly interacts with other drugs. However, enzyme-inducing drugs like carbamazepine, phenytoin, or phenobarbital may decrease the serum concentration of zonisamide.

Contraception, Pregnancy, and Breast Feeding

Zonisamide, unlike older antiepileptic medications, does not accelerate the metabolic rate of the liver. In agreement with a reciprocal effect study, it was shown that the hormonal content and contraceptive protection of the birth control pill were not affected during concurrent administration of zonisamide. Epilepsy minimally increases the risk of birth defects, even without antiepileptic drugs. The risk is not increased while being treated with this antiepileptic medication. Animal experiments have not provided indicators of fetal damage due to zonisamide. However, should you discover that you have become pregnant while on zonisamide, you should not discontinue the medication on your own accord, as this could lead to an increase in frequency of seizures, which could present a greater harm to your baby than zonisamide itself. Consult a specialist immediately, and discuss the further course of action.

We have now thoroughly informed you about the rare but possible side effects of zonisamide. You should be aware that your doctor selected this medication because it currently presents the best possible treatment for your epilepsy, with minimal side effects.

Successful zonisamide therapy is only possible if you take the medication as directed. Only in this way will you avoid large fluctuations of the drug in your blood. Once full dosage has been established and optimal blood levels have been reached, the rate of seizures should go down. If this is not the case, seek the advice of your epilepsy specialist immediately.

INDEX